Rational Root Canal Treatment in Practice

Quintessentials of Dental Practice – 2
Endodontics - 1

Rational Root Canal Treatment in Practice

By
John M Whitworth

Editor-in-Chief: Nairn H F Wilson
Editor Endodontics: John M Whitworth

Quintessence Publishing Co. Ltd.
London, Berlin, Chicago, Copenhagen, Paris, Milan, Barcelona,
Istanbul, São Paulo, Tokyo, New Delhi, Moscow, Prague, Warsaw

British Library Cataloguing in Publication Data

Whitworth, John
   Rational root canal treatment in practice. - (The quintessentials of dental practice)
   1. Root canal therapy
   I. Title II. Wilson, Nairn H. F.
   617.6'342'06

   ISBN 1850970556

Copyright © 2002 Quintessence Publishing Co. Ltd., London

All rights reserved. This book or any part thereof may not be reproduced, stored in a retrieval system, or transmitted in any form or by any means, electronic, mechanical, photocopying, or otherwise, without the written permission of the publisher.

ISBN 1-85097-055-6

Foreword

Endodontics is one of the fastest-growing aspects of everyday clinical practice. Linked to the sustained growth in endodontics is the introduction of many new instruments, materials and techniques. Keeping abreast of these diverse developments and applying them to the best advantage clinically is a challenge for the specialist, let alone the hard-pressed dental practitioner. *Rational Root Canal Treatment in Practice* - Volume 2 of the Quintessentials Series - has been written to help all those practising endodontics to meet this challenge. From anatomical considerations through the "thrill of the fill" and pointers to long-term success, the many complexities of state-of-the-art endodontics are explained and beautifully illustrated in most careful detail. *Rational Root Canal Treatment in Practice* is a valuable volume in the Quintessentials for General Dental Practitioners Series - an outstanding self-contained update for practitioners and students.

Nairn H F Wilson
Editor-in-Chief

Contents

Chapter 1	**Fundamentals of Endodontic Disease**	1
Chapter 2	**Endodontic Symptomology and Immediate Management**	13
Chapter 3	**Preparing for Definitive Treatment**	27
Chapter 4	**Entering the Canal System**	37
Chapter 5	**Entering "Calcified" Systems**	51
Chapter 6	**Creating the Conditions for Periapical Health**	59
Chapter 7	**Preserving the Healing Environment**	87
Chapter 8	**Success and Failure**	111
	Index	123

Chapter 1
Fundamentals of Endodontic Disease

Aim

To describe the fundamental clinical biology of pulp and periapical disease, and lay the foundations for rationally based endodontic treatment.

Outcome

After studying this chapter, the reader should have clear understanding of the role of microbial infection in pulp and periapical disease, and the need for this knowledge to translate into action at each stage of clinical root canal treatment.

An Introduction to Endodontics

Endodontics is the branch of clinical dentistry concerned with the prevention, diagnosis and treatment of diseases of the dental pulp and their sequela. The discipline therefore has a broad scope, encompassing procedures which aim to:
- preserve all or part of the pulp in health (pulp capping and pulpotomy)
- preserve and restore teeth with irreversibly inflamed and necrotic pulps (pulpectomy and root canal treatment)
- preserve and restore teeth with lesions which have failed to respond to root canal treatment, or which were damaged in the course of such treatment (endodontic retreatment and surgery).

In reality, "endodontic treatment" is usually synonymous with "pulpectomy and root canal treatment", an exacting, technical and rapidly developing element of everyday practice, with its emphasis on line, length, and the attainment of a radiographically pleasing root filling. This book will focus almost exclusively on adult root canal treatment and provide a rational framework for the appraisal and safe application of established and emerging clinical methods.

Fundamentals of Endodontic Disease

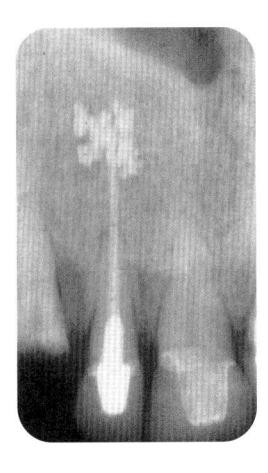

Fig 1-1 Excitement and conviction evaporate into disappointment once again.

The Technological Focus of Root Canal Treatment

Endodontics has never been shy of technology. New systems, devices and materials appear frequently, promising simpler, quicker, more consistent or aesthetically satisfying results. Many of us have invested heavily and repeatedly over the years, convinced and excited by the benefits to follow. Many of us have also known the brief honeymoon of interest and satisfaction which quickly evaporated into disappointment (Fig 1-1); another expensive system relegated to the back of a dark cupboard in preference for an old trusty method, or to be superseded by the next bright hope.

The truth is that most of us find root canal treatment technically challenging, and wish there were simpler, more predictable and more efficient ways to do it. This, combined with a growing demand for tooth preservation, has seen unprecedented growth in world markets for endodontic product, and an insatiable hunger for new and attractively packaged materials and devices. To the dispassionate observer, this may seem to be pure commercial opportunism as we focus on technology and attaining the currently fashionable postoperative "look" rather than returning to the disease process and how it can best be managed.

At the start of a practical handbook on root canal treatment, it is important to ground ourselves in the fundamental biology of the pulp and periapical lesions we wish to prevent and heal. Only then can we rationalise the mechanical stages of treatment and reveal where new and older techniques can optimise operator efficiency and successful outcomes for patients.

Fundamentals of Endodontic Disease

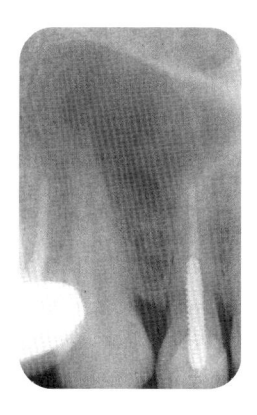

Fig 1-2a Apical periodontitis, an important and common disease in western society.

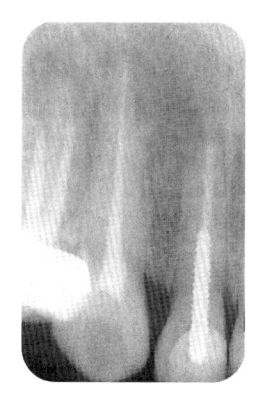

Fig 1-2b Control of aetiological factors allows apical periodontitis to heal.

Laying Foundations: The Basic Biology of Endodontic Disease

Root canal treatment is concerned with preventing and healing apical periodontitis (Fig 1-2a), a disease which affects 40% of over 30s and 62% of over 60s in western society.

Apical periodontitis is important because:
- It causes local pain and morbidity.
- Acute exacerbation can result in serious, potentially life-threatening extension (e.g. facial cellulitis, brain abscess).
- There are growing concerns about the possible systemic consequences of chronic infection and inflammatory lesions associated with teeth.

Apical periodontitis develops by extension of disease in the dental pulp (Fig 1-5). It can be prevented by:
- maintaining pulp health
- managing pulp disease before changes can progress to involve the periapical tissues (Fig 1-3).

Established apical periodontitis is caused by infected material in the pulp canal space and is known to heal predictably if the causative agents can be eliminated and prevented from returning (Fig 1-2a,b).

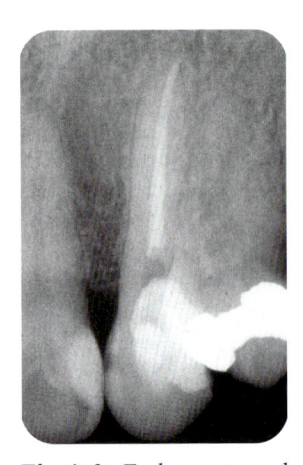

Fig 1-3 Early root canal treatment of a tooth with a dying pulp relieves pain and prevents apical periodontitis from developing.

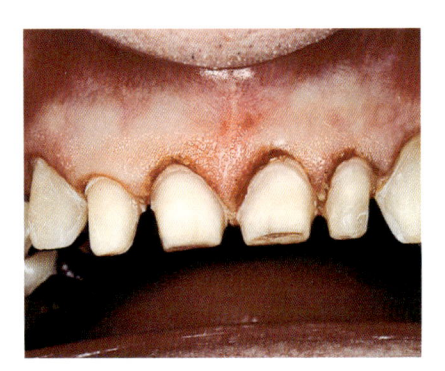

Fig 1-4 Frank exposure of the pulp, or via porous dentine leaves it vulnerable to chemical, physical and above all, microbial injury.

The Aetiology of Pulp Injury and Death

Dentine and pulp are intimately related. In pristine health, the so-called "dentine-pulp complex" lies protected by an impervious layer of enamel and a sound investing periodontium. Breakdown of this protection by caries, operative dentistry or trauma (Fig 1-4) exposes porous, tubular dentine to the oral environment and leaves the pulp vulnerable to chemical, physical and microbial injury. The threat posed by microorganisms is by far the most serious.

The Oral Flora and the Pulp

The virulence of the oral flora was demonstrated in the 1960s, when researchers investigated the effects of pulp exposure in normal and microbe-free animals. Similar observations have been made in subsequent studies on the pulpal irritancy of restorative materials in microbe-free animals and in surface-sealing studies where microbes where kept out of teeth. The overwhelming body of evidence currently supports the view that:
- If microorganisms are kept out of the pulp, it has remarkable capacity to withstand and wall itself off from mechanical and chemical irritation.
- Acids and monomers are less of an issue for pulp health than the percolation of fluids and microorganisms at restoration margins.

- It is the oral flora and their toxins which seriously inflame and kill pulps.

Although a significant number of pulps lose vitality during traumatic events which sever their apical blood supply (sterile, avascular necrosis), most pulp death is still caused by microbial entry following repeated cycles of caries and dental intervention. Almost 20% of crowned teeth, for example, will have non-vital pulps and apical periodontitis within twenty years. This is a sobering reflection as we plan dental care for patients under the age of 60.

Avoiding pulp infection is key to preventing pulp death and apical periodontitis, and must be a fundamental goal of all dentists. However refined we become in root-filling teeth, the best root filling will always be a healthy pulp. A whole volume in this series is devoted to the preservation of pulp health in practice, and another to the management of traumatic injuries.

Dead Pulp Tissue: The Cause of Apical Periodontitis?

As pulp breakdown proceeds from the irritated and infected periphery to the centre, and then apically, canal contents begin to stimulate inflammation in the surrounding tissues (Fig 1-5). Radiographic evidence of bony resorption, the classic diagnostic sign, is one of the consequences.

Historically, textbooks have described stagnation and breakdown of pulp and tissue fluids in the apical part of the canal as major causes of this inflammation. But is this host material sufficiently irritant to provoke and sustain periapical inflammation?

Human studies in the 1970s showed that in teeth devitalised by trauma, only those with infected root canals developed apical periodontitis. Teeth with sterile, necrotic pulps showed no such changes. Primate studies in the 1980s also showed that aseptically devitalising a pulp does not cause apical periodontitis, but if infected saliva is added, apical periodontitis develops rapidly and predictably. Many of us have witnessed such events. Traumatised teeth can remain quiet and symptom free for many months or even years, then suddenly, without serious challenge, they become painful and develop apical periodontitis. The explanation is that the pulp died quietly and aseptically after the trauma. Many years later, the entry of microorganisms (perhaps even just one) to the rich, warm culture medium lying dormant within provided the necessary foreign antigenic challenge to establish and sustain periapical inflammation and the development of a clinically detectable lesion.

Fundamentals of Endodontic Disease

Fig 1-5 The gradual process of pulp death.

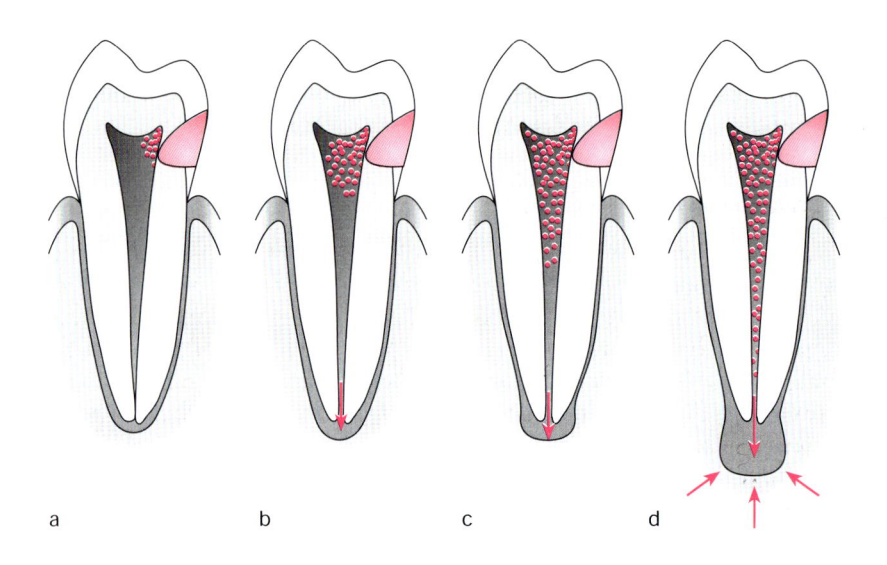

(a) Invasion of the pulp by microorganisms following carious pulp exposure. The pulp mounts a local inflammatory response in an attempt to eliminate or contain the infection. (b,c) Without treatment, inflammation progresses centrally and apically until the whole pulp is dead. Apical inflammation commences early. (d) Established apical periodontitis; an attempt to contain the advance of irritants. Symptoms experienced represent a balance between the contained infection and host defences. The progressive death of the pulp allows successful pulpotomy if caught early.

What does this mean?
- Periapical inflammatory lesions cannot be initiated or sustained by the presence of dead host tissues or stagnant body fluids alone. Foreign antigenic material must be present, and that means microbial infection.
- When we witness apical periodontitis clinically, we are observing the consequences of pulp canal infection.
- Apical periodontitis can only be expected to heal if the causative infection is eliminated and prevented from returning.

The Nature of Root Canal Infection

Whilst the mouth is inhabited by more than 200 microbial species, environmental pressures in the infected root canal typically limit colonisation at any one time to some 4-6 species. Most are strictly anaerobic, though facultative and CO_2-loving (capnophilic) isolates are common.

Specific or Non-specific Infection?

What we do not know is whether apical periodontitis is a response to a critical mass (perhaps very tiny) of any microorganism, or if there must be certain organisms or combinations present for a lesion to develop. Research suggests that a wide range of bacteria can produce periapical inflammation. The apical periodontitis-inducing flora in cases of failed root canal treatment, for example, differs greatly from that of previously untreated cases, and the existence of a "healthy" root canal flora has never been established. For the present, we cannot distinguish the true pathogens from the innocent bystanders, and have no specific drugs to target them. Any root canal infection must therefore be considered unwanted and potentially disease-inducing. Thankfully, our standard methods of disinfection are able to kill most of them.

An Unusual, Inaccessible Infection

The two patients shown in Fig 1-6 are separated by several decades, and present very different clinical histories. We have established that they share a common microbial disease, but neither is able to do anything about it. Their infection is contained in the avascular environment of the necrotic pulp space, inaccessible to host defences, and inaccessible to penetration by any systemic antimicrobial drug.

The only way these patients can be predictably healed of their disease is to:
- extract the affected teeth, including their infected contents, or
- clean their root canal systems as thoroughly, in biological terms, as an extraction would.

Complete periapical healing is a predictable reality in more than 90% of optimally treated cases in which the canal system is properly cleaned and densely sealed against re-infection.

Judging our outcomes is often based on the technical appearance of root fillings (Fig 1-7) — a pleasing white line implying that everything was done cor-

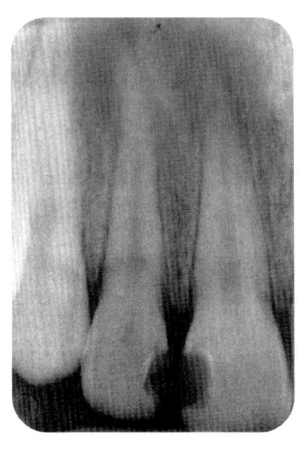

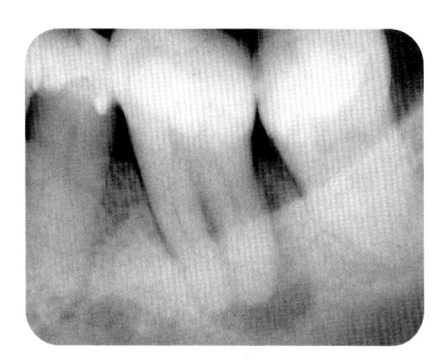

Fig 1-6 Two patients, separated by several decades, share a microbial disease which they are unable to rid themselves of.

rectly. But we should also have an interest to follow up our patients in the longer term for the biological verdict on what we are doing and whether our methods allow our patients to heal.

All of this means that control of infection must underpin all actions and decisions at every clinical stage of root canal treatment from initial evaluation of coronal restorations and caries control, through isolation, finding all of the anatomy, properly cleaning and shaping it, to sealing against new infection. Subsequent chapters will address these technical, clinical stages with due emphasis on rational measures for optimising infection control.

What About the "Therapy-resistant" Lesion?

Clinicians have tried for many years to distinguish periapical lesions which will respond to simple root canal treatment from those which will not. Classically, any lesion with a corticated margin and a diameter of 1cm or more (Fig 1-8) was regarded as a cyst, in need of surgical enucleation. These clinical features may well suggest a cyst, but very many of these lesions are apical pocket cysts (Fig 1-9), which will respond as well to simple root canal treatment as granulomatous chronic inflammatory lesions. Since there is currently no way of differentiating clinically between the apical pocket cyst and the "therapy-resistant" apical true cyst, there is rarely justification for surgical intervention before the outcome of high-quality, routine treatment is known.

Fundamentals of Endodontic Disease

Fig 1-7 An apparently successful root canal treatment. But were infection control measures adequate? Only time will provide the biological verdict.

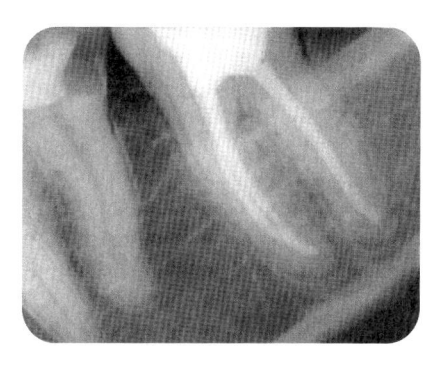

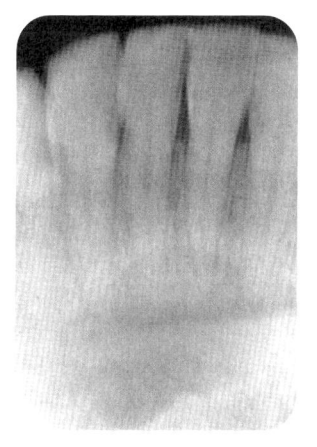

Fig 1-8a A therapy-resistant lesion in need of surgical enucleation?

Fig 1-8b Substantial healing just six months after disinfecting the root canal and sealing the coronal entrance.

Most other failing cases and "therapy-resistant" lesions are easy to explain on infection-control grounds:
- failure to enter all of the anatomy harbouring microorganisms (missed canals)
- failure to use proper methods of cleaning and disinfection (inadequate isolation, enlargement, irrigation)
- failure to prevent reactivation of residual microorganisms (inadequate root filling)
- failure to prevent new infection from the mouth (inadequate coronal seal).

Fundamentals of Endodontic Disease

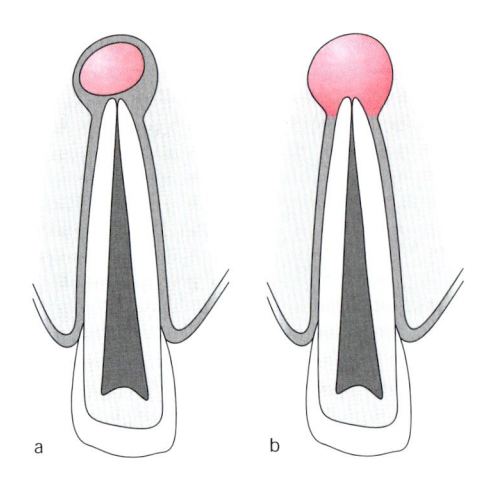

Fig 1-9 Periapical **(a)** true and **(b)** pocket cysts. The pocket cyst with its communication to the canal system will probably heal after simple treatment. Differentiation is impossible with current diagnostic methods.

Rare exceptions include the presence of:
- a disinfectant-resistant flora, such as *Actinomyces* spp or *Enterococcus faecalis*
- an established infection on the external root surface, which cannot be reached by intracanal instruments and disinfectants
- apical impaction of other foreign materials, classically leguminous vegetable matter in teeth left on open drainage for extended periods.

There will, of course, be occasional sinister lesions which may be missed and which fail to respond to root canal treatment. We are healthcare professionals, not root canal therapists, and need to be vigilant for the unusually presenting or behaving lesion at all times. Nevertheless, common lesions are common and should be treated by simple, predictable and minimally invasive methods whenever possible.

Conclusions

- Clinical endodontics can focus too much on the mechanistic and the postoperative appearance of root fillings.
- Our concern as dentists should be the most efficient and effective ways of preventing and healing apical periodontitis, not just making aesthetic root fillings.
- Pulp and periapical disease are caused by microbial infection.
- Successful management of pulp and periapical disease requires attention

to detail in eliminating and preventing the recurrence of microbial infection at every stage of treatment.
- Dentists have a responsibility to audit their biological, healing outcomes and modify their practices accordingly, and to be alert for the occasional non-responding or sinister lesion.

Further Reading

Cox CF, Hafez AA. Biocomposition and reaction of pulp tissues to restorative treatments. Dent Clinics N Amer. 2001;45:31-48.

Dahlen G, Haapasalo M. Microbiology of apical periodontitis. In: Orstavik D, Pitt Ford TR (Eds.) Essential Endodontology: Prevention and Treatment of Apical Periodontitis. Oxford: Blackwell Science, 1998:106-130.

Nair PN. Apical periodontitis: a dynamic encounter between root canal infection and host response. Periodontology 2000. 1997;13:121-148.

Chapter 2
Endodontic Symptomology and Immediate Management

Aim

To describe the characteristics of symptomatic pulpitis and apical periodontitis, and approaches to their diagnosis and immediate clinical management.

Outcome

After studying this chapter, the reader should have a clearer understanding of endodontic symptomology, diagnosis and rational measures for effective immediate management.

Endodontic Emergencies

Endogenous infection from the oral flora presents a threat to everyone with teeth on a disease continuum from niggling pulp inflammation to potentially life-threatening sepsis. Many patients requiring root canal treatment first present with symptoms of pulp or periapical inflammation requiring diagnosis and immediate management. These patients are usually unscheduled, squeezed into an already busy list of appointments, and easy to mismanage under pressure. Even if extraction becomes the definitive outcome, a simple endodontic procedure can often halt the progression of disease and buy pain-free time to reflect on the final plan of care. Well done, it will also provide a valuable foundation for subsequent endodontic treatment.

Immediate management should be based on the surgical principles of:
- identifying the cause by reproducing symptoms
- removing the cause
- securing drainage of any purulent focus
- preventing extension.

This may or may not involve the use of antimicrobial or analgesic drugs, which should not be seen as a way of avoiding proper diagnosis and surgical care.

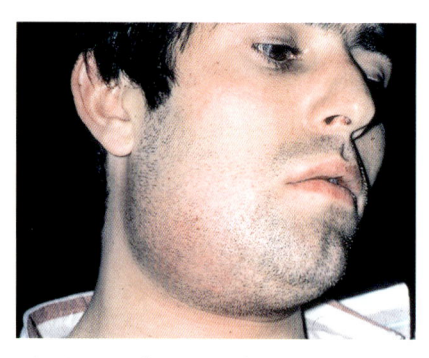

Fig 2-1 What started as an untreated minor niggle.

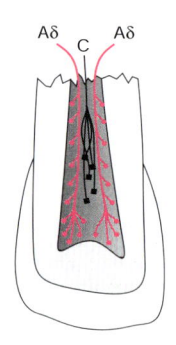

Fig 2-2 Location of predominant sensory pain receptors. Fast-reacting Aδ fibres lie peripherally whilst slow-reacting C fibres reside in the core.

Pulp and periapical infection should not be trivialised and should be treated early and well. Whilst the majority of affluent, dentally aware, fit and healthy individuals probably regard dental sepsis as the stuff of comic cartoons, a significant number of individuals still experience pain and swelling of endodontic origin. Some of these:
- do not have ready access to routine affordable dental care
- are immunocompromised by disease or iatrogenically (e.g. following organ transplantation)
- may be in danger of infection from antibiotic-resistant microorganisms and can be seriously compromised by dental infection (Fig 2-1).

Common scenarios will be considered under the headings:
- Symptomatic pulpitis (reversible and irreversible)
- Symptomatic apical periodontitis (contained and spreading).

Symptomatic Pulpitis

Dental pulps have a rich sensory nerve supply from the trigeminal nerve. Most of the nerve endings are nociceptive, communicating discomfort or pain.

At the periphery of the pulp lie the nerve-endings of Aδ fibres (Fig 2-2), characterised by:
- low threshold of stimulation

- fast reaction and conduction
- communication of sharp, fleeting pain sensation.

These are the fibres stimulated when dentine is exposed to the mouth by gingival recession, traumatic loss of enamel, lost or leaking restorations, or early dental caries.

Pain is usually stimulated by hot, cold or sweet foodstuffs and disappears as soon as the stimulus is withdrawn. A history of Aδ pain usually indicates superficial and minor irritation or inflammation of the pulp; reversible injury which will resolve if the insult can be removed.

More centrally placed are sensory C fibres (Fig 2-2), characterised by:
- high threshold of stimulation
- slow reaction and conduction
- communication of heavy, dull, intense pain, often throbbing in nature.

These are the fibres stimulated by serious inflammation spreading deep into the centre of the pulp. C-fibre pain is often preceded by Aδ pain, and is the classic "toothache". It can be stimulated by hot, cold and sweet foodstuffs, but unlike Aδ pain, it does not disappear immediately after the stimulus is withdrawn, and will often linger for minutes. It can also appear spontaneously, classically waking patients at night when there is no stimulus in the mouth to provoke it. A history of C fibre pain indicates serious and probably irreversible damage to the pulp.

Symptomatic Pulpitis – Diagnostic Challenges

- You cannot see it.

Unlike an inflamed finger, the location and condition of a symptomatic pulp cannot be diagnosed by direct visual inspection. Circumstantial evidence may come from the presence of caries or a lost or leaking restoration, but often the culprit is far from clear.

- The patient cannot locate it.

Pulps have no proprioceptive nerve fibres. Usually symptoms are experienced in a general area on one side of the mouth; sometimes pinpointed by rationalisation or referral to a tooth which was treated or troublesome in the past. Referral between the maxilla and mandible on the same side of the mouth is common (Fig 2-3). The unwary or unduly trusting are easily caught out.

- Pulpal pain must be reproduced.

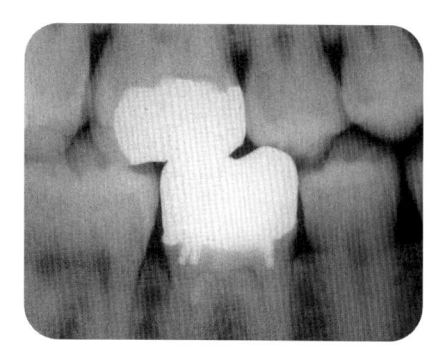

Endodontic Symptomology and Immediate Management

Fig 2-3 Poor pain location. Symptoms were rationalised to a lower first molar which was painful and painfully pulpotomised a decade earlier. The offending tooth was actually the opposing upper first molar.

Ideally, the patient will not have taken analgesics in the hours before presentation, and an appropriate stimulus should be applied. Patients rarely give a history of "pain on electronic stimulation" and the electronic pulp tester has little or no place in diagnosing the location or state of a symptomatic pulp. Thermal challenges should be applied, either cold or hot, and walked in random order from tooth to tooth in an effort to reproduce symptoms. Pulps under large restorations or thick dentine can be difficult to challenge, and ice-sticks (Fig 2-4) provide a reproducible, profound, durable and inexpensive method. Time usually rules out individual tooth isolation and bathing with a jet of kettle-hot water.

Teeth with enamel-dentine cracks and symptomatic pulpitis are often particularly challenging to diagnose, with sporadic, inconsistent histories of thermal sensitivity and pain on chewing, which does not really represent tenderness to percussion. Their pulpal symptoms can often be reproduced by biting on a wedging device (Fig 2-5), which forces crack flexion, movement of dentine fluid and pain. Symptoms are often most profound on release of biting pressure as the displaced cusp recoils rapidly.

Reversible Pulpitis

Reversible pulpitis is characterised by a history and clinical reproducibility of sharp, transient, poorly localised thermal sensitivity (Aδ fibre pain). If the cause is removed, and extension prevented, the pulp should return to health.

Remove the cause
Caries or defective restorations should be removed. If the cause is a crack, its course should be investigated, ideally with transillumination and stains.

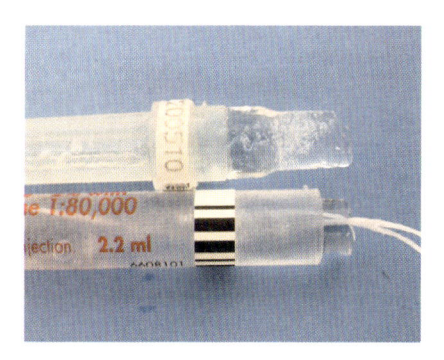

Endodontic Symptomology and Immediate Management

Fig 2-4 Ice-sticks made from local anaesthetic cartridges and floss, or needle sheaths provide an inexpensive, durable and reproducible cold challenge. Used cartridges or sheaths present cross infection risks and should be avoided.

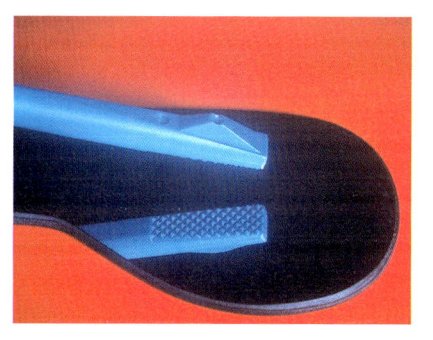

Fig 2-5 Tooth sleuth, one of several commercial wedging devices for the displacement of incomplete tooth fractures and reproduction of pulp sensitivity due to fluid movement in the crack and Aδ nerve stimulation.

Undermined, flexing cusps should be removed for overlay with restorative material.

Prevent extension
The cavity should be sealed, bacteria- and fluid-tight. More than 95% of cases will experience relief from a simple zinc oxide-eugenol cement dressing. It is not currently known if the outcome is better following cavity sealing with a resin bonding agent.

Definitive restoration can be arranged after symptoms have resolved, and the tooth should be monitored for signs and symptoms of irreversible pulpitis or pulp necrosis with apical periodontitis.

Irreversible Pulpitis

Irreversible pulpitis is characterised by a history of provoked and spontaneous dull, heavy and lingering thermal pain which can be reproduced clinically (C fibre pain). Regardless of operative efforts, the pulp cannot return to health, but extension can and should be prevented.

Remove the cause
Caries and defective restorations should be removed under local anaesthesia, before entry into the pulp chamber.

Endodontic Symptomology and Immediate Management

Drain
Occasionally, pulp exposure during initial excavation yields a very satisfying discharge of pus from a pulp abscess, reinforcing a correct diagnosis and bringing substantial pain relief.

Prevent extension
The most reliable way of relieving pain and preventing extension is to remove the entire pulp and thoroughly clean and shape the canal system. In an emergency:
- anaesthetic difficulties
- limitation of time

may rule this out.

Anaesthetic Difficulties

Most failures of local anaesthesia are due to inaccurate deposition or an inadequate dose of anaesthetic agent. In the case of the "hot" pulp, anaesthesia may not reach effective working levels despite profound anaesthesia of related structures. Explanations include changes in the membrane potential of inflammation-associated peripheral nerves, rendering them resistant to anaesthesia, or central heightening of sensory perception. Failed anaesthesia is a major and poorly understood issue in dentistry, and one which continues to reinforce public apprehension of endodontic procedures.

Dealing with anaesthetic difficulties
Approaches to failed anaesthesia include
- increasing the effective dose
- targeting or circumventing alternative routes of innervation
- use of an alternative agent.

Increasing the effective dose may involve repeating an infiltration or block, or delivering it higher (e.g. Akinosi block) but mindful of the toxic limits of the agent in use. In the case of a maxillary molar, infiltrations may be targeted at individual roots (mesiobuccal, distobuccal and palatal), and for mandibular molars, blocking the long buccal nerve and infiltrating beneath the periosteum of the thin lingual plate over the tooth apices may be helpful. Intraosseous injections in the form of:
- periodontal ligament infiltration
- intraseptal infiltration
- delivery though a puncture hole in the buccal cortical plate

may also be potent supplements.

Endodontic Symptomology and Immediate Management

Sometimes it is necessary to infiltrate directly into pulp tissue, which operates by high-pressure concussion of pulpal nerves and is independent of the anaesthetic agent. This transiently painful method demands the good will of the patient, but acts almost immediately to allow rapid entry and removal of pulp tissue.

Whilst lidocaine and epinephrine remains the gold-standard local anaesthetic agent, alternatives, notably articaine, may offer greater penetration in difficult situations.

Limitation of Time

Time often forces a lesser procedure, in order of pain-relieving reliability:
- gross pulp extirpation
- coronal pulp amputation (pulpotomy)
- wide pulpal exposure and dressing.

Pain relief is related more to caries removal and tight sealing of the cavity than to the precise composition of any "obtundent" medication. The antibiotic/steroid preparation Ledermix™ and various setting and non-setting calcium hydroxide preparations are popular in the UK.

Pain relief will be secured in more than 90% of cases provided that something operative is done. Antibiotics alone will offer no relief in the immediate term and have no place in the management of symptomatic pulpitis.

Symptomatic Apical Periodontitis   — around the apical apex

Symptomatic apical periodontitis is characterised by:
- a dead or dying pulp
- pain on chewing or tooth movement
- a pressurised sensation of the tooth rising in its socket
- fine localisation by the patient as the affected periodontal ligament is richly supplied with proprioceptive sensory nerve endings.

New cases arise in teeth with cumulative restorative histories, or which have undergone pulp infection and breakdown after caries or trauma. Many also represent acute exacerbations of painless, chronic lesions signifying a shift in the host/infection balance (Fig 2-6).

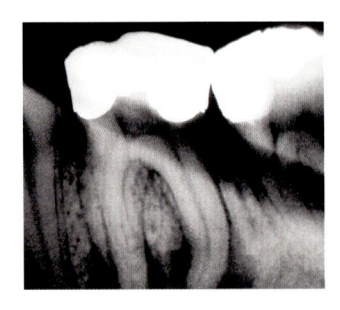

Endodontic Symptomology and Immediate Management

Fig 2-6 Acute exacerbation of a long-standing, silent lesion present on a repeatedly restored and crowned tooth.

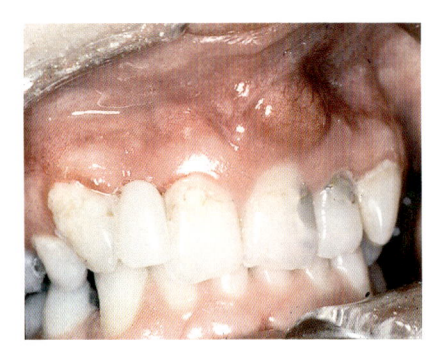

Fig 2-7 Circumscribed swelling in contained acute apical periodontitis. The patient is systemically well.

Symptomatic apical periodontitis is important because of the:
- local pain, swelling and suffering that it causes, and the
- potentially serious consequences of extension.

Contained Symptomatic Apical Periodontitis

In the contained situation, inflammation may be confined within bone (no local swelling), or associated with a circumscribed area of swelling. The patient may have enlarged local lymph nodes but feels generally well and does not have a raised temperature. The offending tooth is identified by:
- the presence of a localised swelling (Fig 2-7)
- negative pulp sensitivity testing. Here the electronic pulp tester adds to the diagnosis, remembering that apical periodontitis can be present in teeth with remnants of living tissue, and that multi-rooted teeth may contain tissue in different states
- tenderness on biting or gentle percussion. Percussion or pressure with a finger tip is often sufficient to provoke a response
- radiographic signs of apical or lateral bony rarefaction.

During immediate treatment, it should be remembered that the infection causing symptoms is contained in the pulp canal of the offending tooth; the periapical changes are a response to this contained infection.

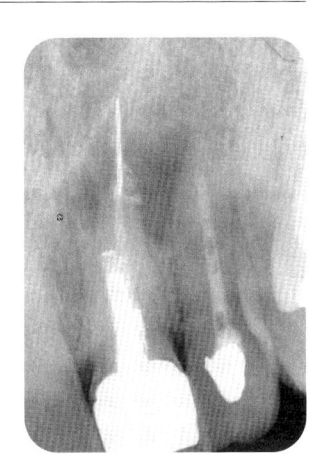

Endodontic Symptomology and Immediate Management

Fig 2-8 Cortical trepanation may be needed to drain and relieve pressure from a painful lesion which cannot be simply liberated through the canal. A rare event in teeth not previously root-treated.

No Soft Tissue Swelling

Remove the cause
Open the tooth under local anaesthesia and rubber dam, clean and irrigate the canals. Ideally the canals should be fully cleaned and shaped.

Drain
Sometimes spontaneous drainage occurs from a pressurised focus of periapical pus. This can be encouraged by apical trepanation with a file no larger than size 25, gently inserted beyond the root-end. There are rare occasions in teeth not previously root treated in which discharge cannot be secured through the canal, and the cortical plate must be punctured with a bur to release pressure and secure discharge (Fig 2-8).

Prevent extension
Extension is best prevented by thorough canal preparation, but this may be limited in an emergency situation. An antimicrobial calcium hydroxide or steroid-antibiotic paste may help to control intracanal infection, sealed in place with a cotton pledget to guard against blockage of canal entrances, and a 3mm thickness of well-adapted cement dressing. Special care should be taken to avoid the presentation of cotton wool fibres at the cavity margins, which may wick infected saliva into the tooth.

Endodontic Symptomology and Immediate Management

Supportive therapy
Standard measures can be supplemented to aid pain relief and recovery:
- Relieve the occlusion. There is no surer way to exacerbate periapical pain than to leave an extruded tooth in heavy occlusion.
- Ensure adequate nutrition and hydration. Patients with toothache frequently neglect to eat and drink properly.
- Analgesia. Pain relief usually follows rapidly once pressure has been relieved, but patients with persistent discomfort should be advised to use normal non-steroidal inflammatory drugs if needed. Dissimilar agents such as paracetamol (acetaminophen) and ibuprofen can be taken regularly at staggered intervals to avoid troughs in analgesia, and without risk of toxicity associated with over-use of individual agents.
- Antibiotics. Antibiotics should not be used as a means of avoiding surgical intervention. They should not be prescribed if the tooth can be opened and cleaned, if the patient is generally well and not immunocompromised, and if it will be possible to make contact with them during the following days. Patients at risk of infective endocarditis should be covered for acute endodontic procedures of this sort.

Local Soft Tissue Swelling

Management follows the same pattern as described for symptomatic apical periodontitis with no soft tissue swelling. It should again be emphasised that despite the presence of a soft tissue lesion, the cause is still infection inside the offending tooth.

Additional considerations
Open drainage
Drainage through the root canal may occasionally persist for many minutes. This can usually be dealt with by asking the patient to sit in a quiet and private area for a few minutes with a disposable cup as the tooth continues to discharge. Gentle sucking on the tooth may help. Whilst there is little evidence that leaving teeth open for drainage has a serious impact on eventual healing, this practice can be associated with intractable foreign body responses to food debris impacted beyond the root-apex and anecdotally with refractory infection. Leaving teeth open for drainage is an occasional, extreme measure, continued for no more than 24 hours before canal debridement and closure.

Soft-tissue incision
Not all pus will drain through a root canal, even with apical trepanation and

gentle external pressure to encourage it. In these situations, the fluctuant soft tissue swelling should be incised under block or distant infiltration local anaesthesia, or following topical anaesthesia with gel or a jet of ethyl chloride. The most dependent point of the swelling should be punctured with a scalpel and due regard for local anatomical structures. Discharge can be assisted by blunt dissection with a haemostat, which is introduced closed, opened in the wound, and withdrawn open to avoid trapping tissues. There is little evidence to support the use of rubber drains for intraoral sites, which can be encouraged to remain open and discharge with frequent warm salt water mouthwashes.

Antibiotics and analgesics
Drugs are seldom indicated for well, immunocompetent patients after drainage and elimination of infection. However, there may be occasions where satisfactory drainage is not secured (e.g. in the region of the mental nerve), and the use of antibiotics is supported.

Prescribing is empirical, with the emphasis on short, sharp courses and daily patient contact or review.

Empirical prescribing (contained apical periodontitis)

    3g amoxicillin orally, loading dose; PLUS further 3g amoxicillin orally 8 h later, or 250mg qds for 5 days

Penicillin-allergic patients should receive:

    erythromycin 250mg or clindamycin 150mg qds for 5 days

Either of these regimes can be supplemented by metronidazole 200mg tds for 5 days, if monitoring and further surgical intervention fail to demonstrate satisfactory progress.

Spreading Symptomatic Apical Periodontitis

In the advanced stages of spreading symptomatic apical periodontitis, microorganisms may migrate from the root canal system and track through the fascial spaces of the head and neck, occasionally causing serious and life-threatening disorders such as Ludwig's angina, mediastinitis, cavernous sinus thrombosis or brain abscess. These patients are often systemically unwell and have an elevated temperature (Fig 2-9).

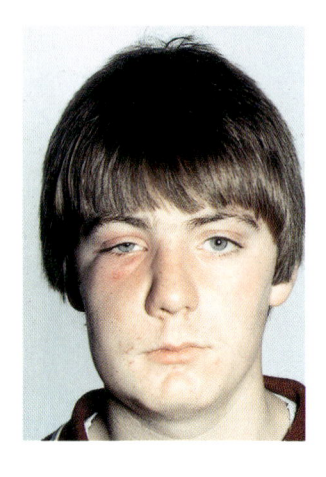

Endodontic Symptomology and Immediate Management

Fig 2-9 An unwell patient with spreading infection of endodontic origin. In the pre-antibiotic era, the prognosis may have been grave.

The primary focus of the infection is again the infected contents of a tooth. Endodontic infections should ideally be diagnosed and properly treated before this stage, when management along conventional guidelines may be difficult.

Remove the cause
In patients with serious, spreading infection, mouth opening is often limited and it can be very difficult to diagnose, open and manage infection in the offending tooth. Extraction can be equally difficult.

Drain
Spreading infections are difficult to drain until they have become localised, with no fluctuation to incise and the temptation to incise into tissues whose surgical anatomy is not frequently remembered.

Prevent extension
Extension should be prevented by the empirical prescription of high-dose antibiotics, the avoidance of warm facial compresses which may promote extension through the facial tissues, and the avoidance of physical exertion.

Empirical prescribing (spreading infections)

> 3g amoxicillin orally, loading dose; PLUS amoxicillin 500mg orally qds for 5 days; PLUS metronidazole 200-400mg orally tds for 5 days.

Penicillin-allergic patients should receive:

> erythromycin 500mg qds for 5 days or
> clindamycin 300mg qds for 5 days; PLUS metronidazole 200-400mg orally tds for 5 days.

Supportive therapy includes adequate fluid and nutritional intake, and at least daily contact to assess progress.

Most lesions will localise within days to become contained and amenable to pulp canal entry and incision and drainage of a circumscribed soft tissue fluctuance. Some will not.

Warning Signs which Indicate Immediate Referral to Hospital
- dysphagia
- respiratory difficulty
- raised/stiff floor of mouth
- soft palate involvement
- impared vision/eye movement
- hoarseness
- lethargy
- impaired consciousness
- dehydration/malnutrition
- temperature of 39ºC.

Hospital admission will allow
- empirical, followed by specific intravenous antibiotics
- airway protection
- fluid and nutritional support
- drainage of affected sites and removal of the source
- close monitoring.

Mercifully, such serious events are currently rare, though it should never be forgotten that the process leading to this end begins with the entry of oral microorganisms to the pulp space.

Conclusions
- Symptomatic pulpitis and apical periodontitis should not be trivialised.

- Disease is usually caused by microorganisms contained within the pulp space.
- Diagnosis is based on reproducing presenting symptoms.
- Immediate care is based on established surgical principles with little or no role for antimicrobial drugs in healthy, non-compromised patients.
- Lesions should be treated early to minimise the risk of more serious extension which can occasionally be life-threatening.

Further Reading

Dumsha TC, Gutmann JL. Problems in managing endodontic emergencies. In: Gutmann JL, Dumsha TC, Lovdahl PE, Hovland EJ (Eds.) Problem Solving in Endodontics. 3rd ed. St Louis: Mosby, 1997:229-252.

Walton RE, Reader AW. Local anesthesia. In: Walton RE, Torabinejad M (Eds.) Principles and Practice of Endodontics. 3rd ed. Philadelphia: Saunders, 2002:99-117.

Walton RE, Torabinejad M. Diagnosis and treatment planning. In: Walton RE, Torabinejad M (Eds.) Principles and Practice of Endodontics. 3rd ed. Philadelphia: Saunders, 2002:49-70.

Chapter 3
Preparing for Definitive Treatment

Aim
To introduce important issues in the assessment of a tooth for definitive root canal treatment and describe preparatory measures including the need for local anaesthesia, occlusal adjustment and simple methods of rubber dam isolation.

Outcome
After studying this chapter, the reader should have a clear view of general and local issues in planning definitive root canal treatment and understand the value of rational preparatory measures including rubber dam isolation.

The immediate management of symptomatic teeth was described in Chapter 2. In subsequent chapters, it will be assumed that acute symptoms have been controlled.

Not Everything That Can Be Root Treated Should Be
Current techniques make it possible to access and root fill just about any tooth, but that does not mean that all damaged teeth should be. Root canal treatment must never be an isolated technical exercise; it is simply a means of preserving teeth for restoration within the context of a holistic treatment plan.

The following questions should be asked:
- What is the role of the tooth within a broader plan of care?
- Is it restorable?
- Can I control infection in it?
- Are there any additional factors which weigh the case for root canal treatment or extraction?

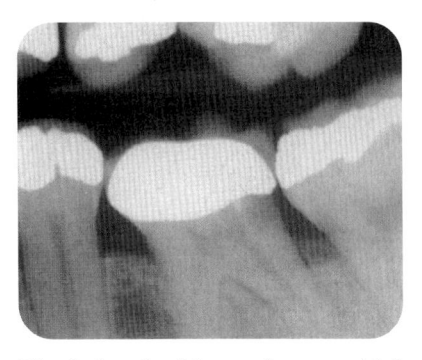

Fig 3-1a Is this tooth restorable? Should the restoration and caries be removed before making any promises?

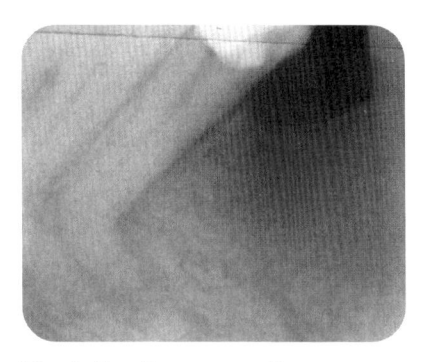

Fig 3-1b Can you really expect to control infection in this tooth?

Decisions should be based on clinical and medical history, clinical examination and recent, good-quality radiographs as well as patient aspirations and finances. Even if large extraoral films have been exposed for general planning, small intraoral films are often justified for greater detail. Images should be projected as near to actual size as possible by the use of a paralleling device (Fig 6-9).

What is the Role of the Tooth Within a Broader Plan?

Questions might include:
- Is there merit in sacrificing a molar as part of a planned shortened dental arch approach to the mouth?
- Would preservation of a last standing molar be highly advantageous in avoiding a free-end saddle denture?
- Would that grossly carious or periodontally compromised canine serve well if the root canal was treated as an overdenture abutment, even if its likely lifespan were limited?

Is the Tooth Restorable?

Patients should not be made promises before teeth have been properly explored and facts are known. Often that is more than just a thorough clinical and radiographic examination (Fig 3-1a).

Defective restorations should be removed and caries ruthlessly excavated, ensuring that the amelodentinal junction is sound at every point, and that

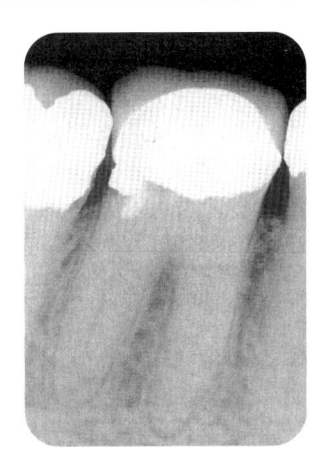

Fig 3-2 Removal of this defective crown revealed grossly carious, rubbery coronal tissue.

the entire crown is fee from soft, infected dentine. Caries is regularly found hiding under radiodense crowns, the only clue being a clinically or radiographically defective margin (Fig 3-2). If there is any doubt, it is better to remove the restoration and caries, discover that the tooth is unrestorable and make alternative plans, rather than fight through infected caries in an effort to preserve a tooth with rubber-like coronal tissue which will fail expensively before long.

Teeth with cracks should be examined by transillumination, with stains and wedging devices to ensure that there are no:
- oblique marginal fractures extending deeply below the alveolar crest and which will be impossible to restore
- prominent and mobile fractures extending through furcal areas or down the roots of anterior teeth.

Such cases have a compromised prognosis, even with contemporary bonding techniques, and the patient should be made aware of this fact before decisions are made.

If a tooth is unrestorable for any reason, root canal treatment is a waste of time, effort, money, patient confidence and goodwill. It is best avoided from the outset.

Can I Control Infection in It?

Endodontic success is synonymous with the elimination of root canal infection. If a tooth cannot be isolated from the oral flora with a well-fitting rubber dam, is it restorable, and can there be adequate infection control for long-term success?

Canal number, position, calcification and curvature may also present local, technical challenges and raise questions:
- Can I successfully enter this canal system and eliminate the infection (Fig 3-1b)?
- Should I recommend referral or extraction, or should I offer to treat after advising the patient on potential difficulties, and compromise?

Matters may be further complicated in patients with limited opening. Arbitrary measurements of acceptable opening are not helpful; the space necessary will depend on the position and angulation of the tooth, the hand size and techniques employed by the practitioner.

Interappointment infection control should be considered in planning. Will a temporary post crown, for example, provide satisfactory protection against reinfection in a decoronated anterior tooth, or should a temporary partial overdenture be made to cover the sealed root face until definitive obturation and restoration are possible? Alternatively, should the care be planned to complete root canal treatment and a sealing coronal post and core at a single visit (Fig 8-5)?

Additional Factors Which May Weight Decision-making

Medical considerations
There are few medical contraindications for root canal treatment. Teeth of doubtful prognosis are probably best removed in patients about to undergo radiotherapy to the jaws or who are seriously immunocompromised.

Conversely, root canal treatment carries a lower risk of bleeding, bacteraemia and local tissue damage than extraction and may be positively indicated in patients with:
- bleeding disorders
- increased risk of infective endocarditis
- history of radiotherapy to the head and neck.

American Heart Association guidelines explicitly list root canal treatment as a low-risk procedure, requiring no antimicrobial prophylaxis, provided that instruments remain within the tooth.

Preparing for Definitive Treatment

weakened molar

damaging wedging forces

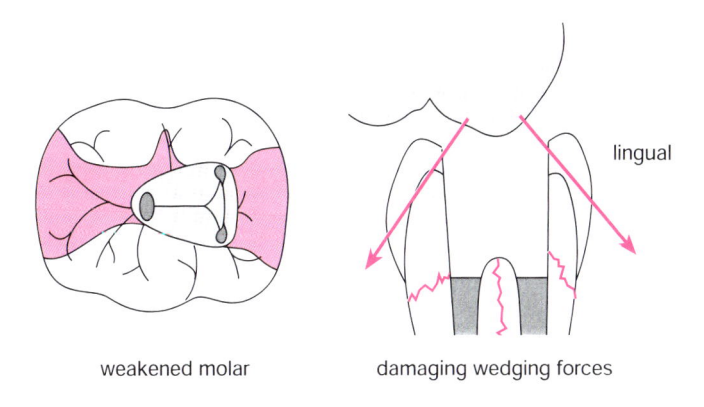

Fig 3-3 The dangers of wedging forces in a weakened posterior tooth.

Socio-economic considerations
Decision-making is often critically influenced by the environment in which the dentist works, and the financial status, attitude to dental care and will of the patient.

Local Anaesthesia

Subject to patient consent, teeth should aways be anaesthetised for root canal treatment. Even if a tooth has a periapical radiolucency or the canal system has been opened before, there is no guarantee of comfort. Rubber dam isolation may also demand soft tissue anaesthesia. Better to be confident and comfortable than to undermine confidence and disrupt treatment by stopping mid-procedure to administer pain relief.

There is no convincing evidence that patients will reliably act as "apex locators" in the absence of local anaesthesia and there are no real advantages to be gained. Problems of satisfactory local anaesthesia were considered in Chapter 2.

Occlusal Adjustment

Premolars and molars which have lost marginal ridges are especially vulnerable to vertical fracture after coronal access (Fig 3-3). It is also recognised

that occlusal prematurity is a principal cause of discomfort following canal instrumentation; a little apical inflammation can make the tooth rise in its socket to become proud in the occlusion, and a vicious cycle commences. Unless there are special and over-riding occlusal considerations, it is wise routinely to:
- reduce the cusp tips of posterior teeth by 1-2mm before root canal treatment
- plan an immediate cuspal-coverage restoration, even as simple as a composite resin or amalgam to protect the tooth after treatment. Better to sacrifice a little tissue in a controlled way than to suffer catastrophic, unplanned loss at a later date.

Particularly vulnerable teeth can be supported with a well-fitting orthodontic band or copper ring.

Rubber Dam Isolation

Medico-legally, rubber dam isolation is mandatory for all endodontic procedures. Its many advantages make it an indispensable aid, and the friend of anyone wishing to work quickly, safely, and with adequate infection control. Rubber dam isolation:
- excludes saliva and the oral flora from the canal system
- protects the mouth and oropharynx from instruments and sodium hypochlorite
- retracts intrusive soft tissues
- improves patient comfort
- reduces treatment time.

Root canal treatment can be difficult enough without adding limited visibility in a wet, slippery, mobile environment. The fewer teeth isolated, the easier it is to apply and the fewer places it has to leak. Single tooth isolation is the norm and an extensive array of equipment is unnecessary.

Clamp selection

Detailed prescription of clamp patterns for specific teeth is not helpful. A clamp should provide stable, four-point contact below the maximum bulbosity of the tooth to be isolated (Fig 3-4). A small range of clamps, available in standard kit form, is effective for most situations (Fig 3-5). Incisor, "butterfly" clamps are available for anterior teeth, but it is often possible simply to secure the dam with a slip of rubber or a Wedjet® (Hygenic Corporation) (Fig 3-8a,b).

Preparing for Definitive Treatment

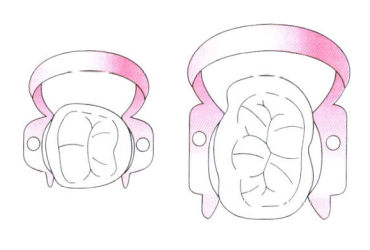

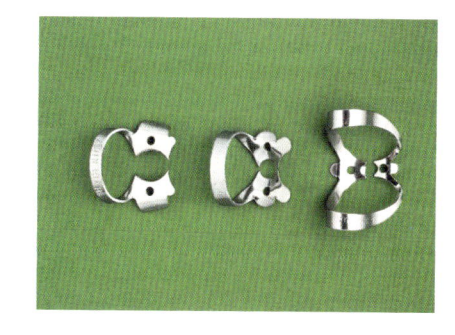

Fig 3-4 Stable, four-point clamp contact beneath the maximum bulbosity.

Fig 3-5 A standard kit containing molar, premolar and butterfly clamps.

Applying the dam
It is usually sufficient to punch a single hole somewhere near the centre of the sheet of rubber (Fig 3-6a). Winged clamps then allow the rubber to be attached to the clamp before it is carried to the mouth (Fig 3-6b). The tooth to be isolated is carefully visualised through the hole, and the clamp slid down in contact with the buccal and lingual surfaces to engage natural undercuts (Fig 3-6c). Alternatively, a winged or wingless clamp can be applied first, before stretching a rather larger hole over the clamp.

The dam should be detached from the wings of the clamp and checked for close adaptation around the tooth (Fig 3-6d). Some practitioners take the additional measure of flossing the rubber through contact points for better proximal adaptation.

However it is secured, the critical issue is that the dam seals. If there is any sign of fluid entry, or even if there is not, a proprietary rubber dam caulking paste, such as Ultradent OraSeal® (Fig 3-7a) or Cavit should be piped around the tooth to provide a tight seal. OraSeal® sticks to moist mucosal surfaces and foams up to fill in gaps even when the dam is not very well adapted (Fig 3-7b). In this way a securely fixed, well-sealing dam can be placed quickly and reliably without getting bogged down in the finer details of technique and component selection. It does not have to be difficult or complicated.

For the fragile or decoronated tooth, a slit dam can be used. A slit dam isolation of a decoronated incisor is shown in Fig 3-8a. A hole was punched for the teeth either side of the damaged tooth. The holes were then joined with

Preparing for Definitive Treatment

Fig 3-6 Application of the dam.

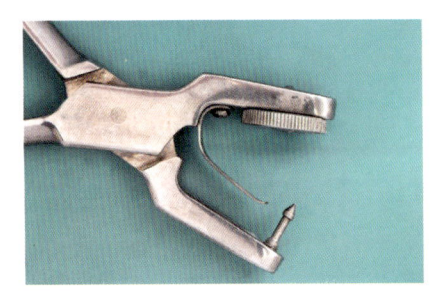

Fig 3-6a A hole punched close to the centre of the dam.

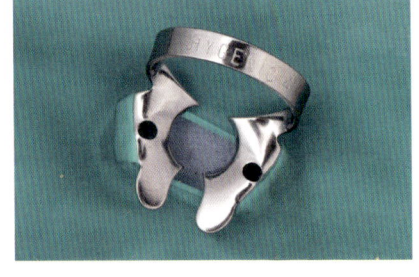

Fig 3-6b Dam engaged on the wings.

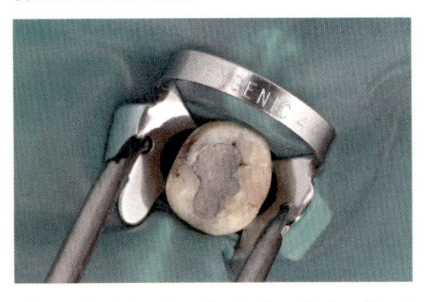

Fig 3-6c Tooth to be isolated visualised through the hole and the jaws of the clamp slid to engage undercuts.

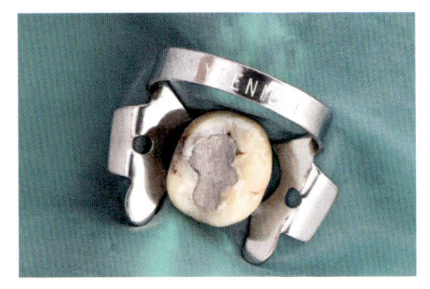

Fig 3-6d Close adaptation of the dam after disengagement of the wings.

Fig 3-7 Dam caulk.

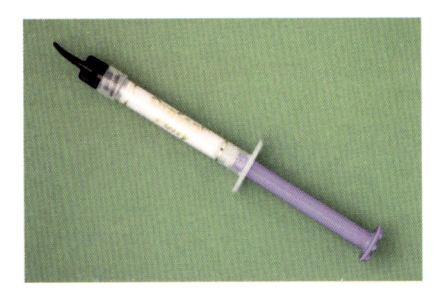

Fig 3-7a OraSeal® dam caulk.

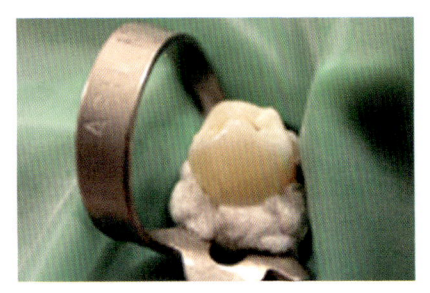

Fig 3-7b OraSeal® sticks and foams up to provide a tight seal.

34

Preparing for Definitive Treatment

Fig 3-8 Slit dam applications. In both cases, the dam is secured anteriorly with a Wedjet®. OraSeal® plugs the gaps.

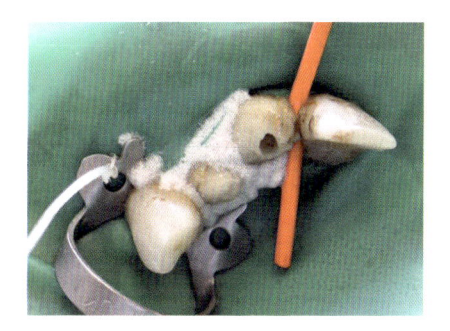

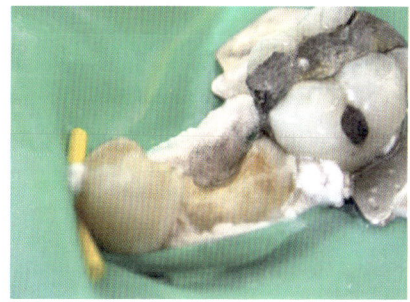

Fig 3-8a Fragile anterior teeth.   **Fig 3-8b** Fragile posterior tooth.

scissors to form a slit. The rubber self-retained after knifing through contact points. This can be supplemented with clamps, a Wedjet® or a small slip of rubber cut from the dam if needed. OraSeal® was applied liberally to seal any deficiencies. Sodium hypochlorite was employed as always without fear or complaint from the patient, and no saliva seepage was noted.

A similar scenario for a damaged posterior tooth is shown in Fig 3-8b. In this case, the distal molar was clamped and the rubber secured mesially with a Wedjet®. OraSeal® again completed the isolation. Even bridgework is no barrier to this simple approach.

Dentists should not be put off by rubber dam. It is a jewel in endodontic practice, and can be applied in most cases with the help of a caulking agent. For those out of the habit of using rubber dam, it is wise to invest in a basic kit, and practise first on a model to build confidence.

Teeth should be isolated from the outset unless there is concern about loss of long-axis orientation during access.

Conclusions

- Not all teeth that can be root treated should be. Even teeth treated with a simple endodontic procedure for pain relief should be properly appraised within a broader plan of care before definitive root canal treatment.

- Due consideration should be given to the fundamentals of infection control in planning and preparing for treatment.
- Sealing rubber dam isolation is mandatory for endodontic care. This does not need to be complicated or time consuming.

Further Reading

Dajani AS, Taubert KA, Wilson W, Bolger AF, Bayer A, Ferrieri P, Gewitz MH, Shulman ST, Nouri S, Newburger JW, Hutto C, Pallasch TJ, Gage TW, Levison ME, Peter G, Zuccaro G Jr. Prevention of bacterial endocarditis. Recommendations by the American Heart Association. (Review) Circulation 1997; 96:358-366.

Glickman GN, Pileggi R. Preparation for treatment. In: Cohen S, Burns RC (Eds.) Pathways of the Pulp. 8th ed. St Louis: Mosby, 2002:103-144.

Scott GL. Isolation. In: Walton RE, Torabinejad M (Eds.) Principles and Practice of Endodontics. 3rd ed. Philadelphia: Saunders, 2002:118-129.

Chapter 4
Entering the Canal System

Aim
To describe the importance of coronal access for effective and efficient management of endodontic infection, and provide clinical guidance for safely uncovering and refining access to the canals of permanent teeth.

Outcome
After studying this chapter, the reader should understand the relevance of dental anatomy in defining access outline, the value of investing time in carefully refining coronal access, and be more conversant with some helpful tools for accessing routine cases.

Access – The Foundation of Success
Managing endodontic infection is a sequential process (Fig 4-1). The consecutive stages of coronal access, root canal preparation, canal obturation and coronal seal build on each other to win success. Coronal access lies at the foundation, and aims to:
- fully unroof the chamber to clean infected and decomposing tissue from all of its pulp horns and ramifications
- uncover the coronal entrances of all root canals which need to be cleaned of soft tissue and infection
- allow simple, unstressed flight-paths for the safe, efficient and controlled use of instruments in the canal system
- preserve as much coronal tooth tissue as possible compatible with these aims. No matter how nice the final radiographic appearance of the root filling, a radical access cavity compromises long-term restorability and does our patients no favours.

Faced with exciting options for canal preparation and obturation, coronal access can be overlooked as a dreary - if sometimes stressful - precursor to be dispensed with quickly before the main event. In fact, coronal access holds the key to success and rewards those who check and refine their preparation before racing to the next stage.

Entering the Canal System

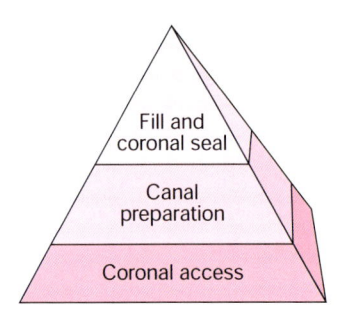

Fig 4-1 The pyramid of endodontic treatment. Everything builds on coronal access.

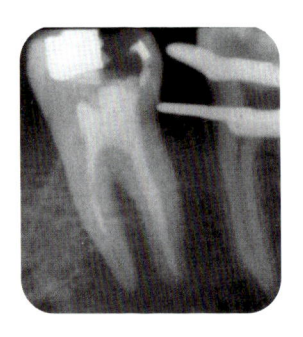

Fig 4-2 A poor root filling and unpredictable bridge abutment, but where did the fatal problem arise?

A lower molar, well treated in the distal canal, but with a short and inadequate root filling mesially is shown in Fig 4-2. In haste to get on, the chamber was not inspected to identify and remove the mesial part of the roof. Instruments fell straight and stress-free into the wide distal canal but the flight path of instruments to the mesial was from the distal, more difficult and frustrating (Fig 4-3a). Advancing under great and unnecessary flexion, the files started to straighten, cutting into the mesial walls to create steps or ledges (Fig 4-3a) which deepened with every exasperated action. The canals were cleaned short, filled short, and the tooth now has a guarded prognosis.

How long might it have taken to remove the mesial pulp chamber roof, provide a simpler, stress-free flight path and win the case with little or no frustration (Fig 4-3b)? We cannot do anything about natural root curvatures, but we can deliver instruments to them in a stress-free, straight line. Access holds the key if we are to avoid rolling problems into the following stages.

Designing Coronal Access – Knowing the Anatomy and Where to Cut

Rational unroofing demands that we know where the pulp is.

Entering the Canal System

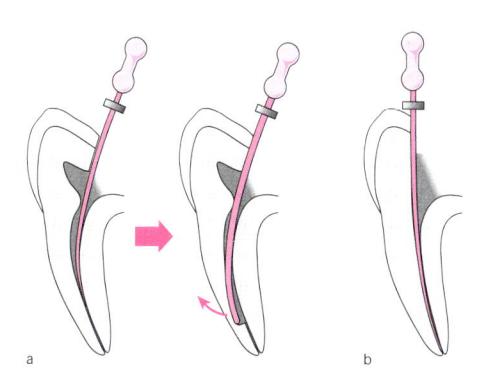

Fig 4-3(a) Difficult flight-path from the distal to find the mesial canal orifices. Instrument recoil results in a ledge which may be impossible to bypass. Dentine mud may occlude the canal below. **(b)** The development of a proper flight-path reduces stress on the instrument and operator.

Guidance is available from:
- classical illustrations in standard texts
- undistorted pre-operative radiographs
- direct visual inspection of the opened chamber.

Idealised pulp anatomy and outline forms for coronal access to sound or soundly restored permanent teeth are shown in Figs 4-4, 4-6 and 4-8. In reality, many teeth presenting for access are far from sound, with caries and defective restorations to be removed, and a large pulpal exposure as the initial entry point. Even here, classical outlines help to rationalise the direction of cutting to develop good access from an unplanned initial opening.

Classic Cavity Outlines

Maxillary central incisors (Fig 4-4a)
Typical length: 23.5mm
Number of canals: 1
Basic access outline: triangular with apex at cingulum.
The coronal pulp is shaped like a fishtail, with mesial and distal pulp horns rising at the lateral limits. A circular access may find the often large canal, but will not properly unroof the pulp horns. Infection will be harboured, and the tooth may discolour as the retained tissue breaks down. For good straight-line access, the preparation will often graze into the incisal edge, but

Fig 4-4 Buccolingual and occlusal views of permanent teeth showing classical pulp anatomy, canal position and access cavity outline.

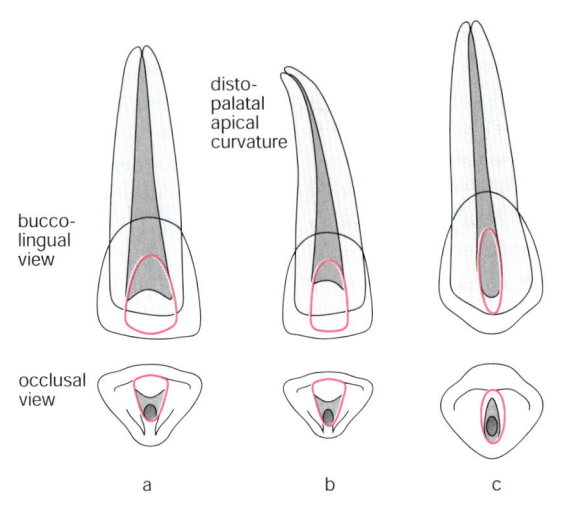

Fig 4-4(a) Maxillary central incisor. **(b)** Maxillary lateral incisor. **(c)** Maxillary canine.

should not extend far labially to create an aesthetic compromise. With age, the pulp narrows mesiodistally and retreats cervically. Access in this case may commence lower on the crown, and be less flared mesiodistally.

Maxillary lateral incisors (Fig 4-4b)
Typical length: 22.5mm
Number of canals: 1
Basic access outline: triangular with apex at cingulum.
A smaller version of the central incisor, lateral incisors catch out the unwary who assume that the root is straight and fail to notice the marked disto-palatal curvature which is almost always present in the apical 2-3mm. Many are ledged or perforated at that point (Fig 4-5), and initial negotiation to the canal terminus often requires precurving the apical 2-3mm of small, flexible instruments (Fig 5-11).

Maxillary canines (Fig 4-4c)
Typical length: 26.5mm
Number of canals: 1
Basic access outline: oval buccolingually.

Entering the Canal System

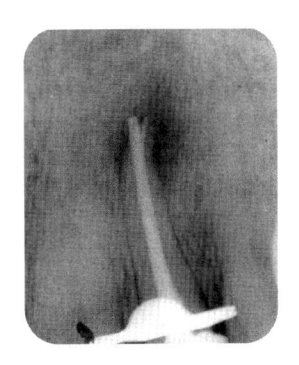

Fig 4-5 A common event in the maxillary lateral incisor. Most have a marked disto-palatal curvature in the apical third.

Maxillary canines have only one pulp horn, lying centrally, so there is no need to flare access mesiodistally. When the pulp is large, a circular access may be excessively wide mesiodistally, but fail to unroof the pulp horn. As the coronal pulp retreats centrally and cervically with age, the outline may be more central and circular.

Maxillary premolars (Fig 4-6a,b)
Typical length: 21mm
Number of canals: first premolar – usually 2; second premolar – usually 1
Basic access outline: oval buccolingually.
Maxillary premolar pulps are narrow and fissure-like mesiodistally, but broad from the buccal to the lingual pulp horns. A mid-occlusal circular access will fail to unroof the pulp horns, and may cause a buccal or lingual canal to be missed.

Maxillary molars (Fig 4-6c,d)
Typical length: 21mm
Number of canals: mesiobuccal root: usually 2
distobuccal root: usually 1
palatal root: usually 1
Basic access outline: triangular, placed mesial to the transverse oblique ridge, with the apex palatally.
The commonest issues in accessing maxillary molars are:
- failure to extend and refine properly for straight-line entry to the major mesiobuccal canal (see later in this chapter for cavity refinements), and
- failure to locate a second mesiobuccal canal which is present in over 60% of cases.

Entering the Canal System

Fig 4-6 Buccolingual and occlusal views of permanent teeth showing classical pulp anatomy, canal position and access cavity outline.

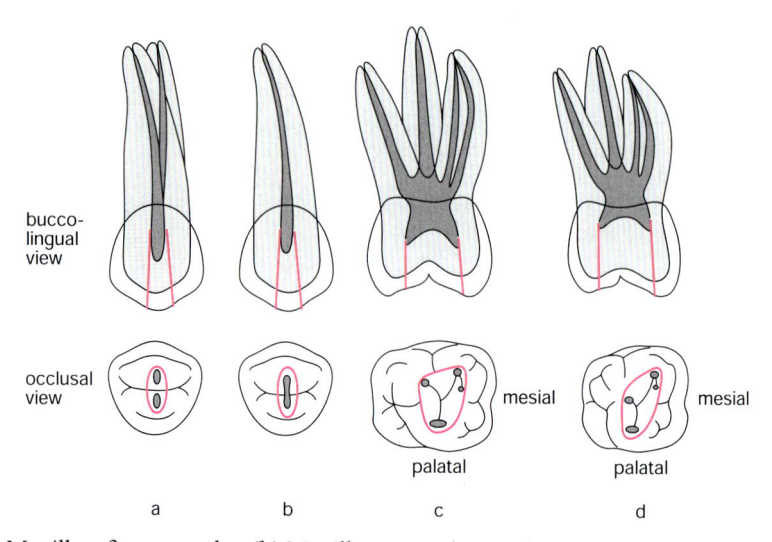

(a) Maxillary first premolar. **(b)** Maxillary second premolar. **(c)** Maxillary first molar. **(d)** Maxillary second molar.

The sectioned roots of an extracted maxillary first molar are shown in Fig 4-7. Notice that the distobuccal and palatal roots are generally circular in cross section. Knowing that dentine is laid down concentrically, it is no surprise that they contain one canal. Although similar looking on a buccolingual radiograph, the mesiobuccal root is quite different in section. It would be surprising if a root of such buccopalatal width did not contain two canals and even a web of tissue between them.

The second mesiobuccal canal is not always easy to locate, but it usually lies just mesial to a line joining the major mesiobuccal and palatal canal entrances. It may be possible to probe it with a long DG16 explorer, but it is usually necessary to run along the mesial chamber floor with a small long-shanked bur or ultrasonic tip (Figs 5-7, 5-9) to uncover the entrance.

The palatal canal may also have surprises; usually appearing straight on the preoperative radiograph, it will often curve markedly towards the buccal.

In maxillary second and third molars, the distobuccal orifice often lies closer to the centre of the tooth than in first molars (Fig 4-6d).

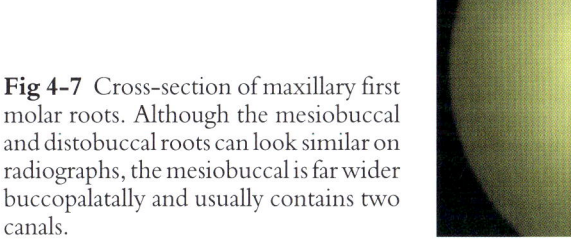

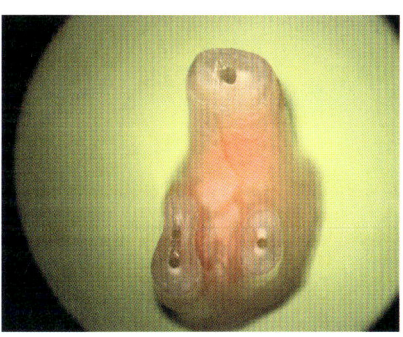

Fig 4-7 Cross-section of maxillary first molar roots. Although the mesiobuccal and distobuccal roots can look similar on radiographs, the mesiobuccal is far wider buccopalatally and usually contains two canals.

Mandibular incisors (Fig 4-8a)
Typical length: 21mm
Number of canals: 1; 2 in approximately 30%
Basic access outline: a narrow triangle, with its apex at the cingulum
Lower incisors are some of the most challenging teeth to access, often with complex anatomy, and little margin for error. The triangular access reflects mesial and distal pulp horns, and extension into the cingulum is often needed to identify the lingual canal. The incisal edge is again just grazed for straight line access.
In teeth where an extracoronal restoration is planned, there may be advantage in accessing more directly through the incisal to preserve the lingual wall and cingulum which will be important for crown retention.

Mandibular canines (Fig 4-8b)
Typical length: 23.5mm
Number of canals: 1; 2 in approximately 30%.
Basic access outline: oval buccolingually.
A smaller version of the maxillary canine coronally, but often with a second, lingual root canal which is uncovered by extension into the cingulum.

Mandibular premolars (Fig 4-8c)
Typical length 21mm
Number of canals: usually 1
Basic access outline: oval bucco lingually.
The coronal pulp is often wider mesiodistally than that of maxillary premolars. Access is often a slightly wider oval to reflect this.

Fig 4-8 Buccolingual and occlusal views of permanent teeth showing classical pulp anatomy, canal position and access cavity outline.

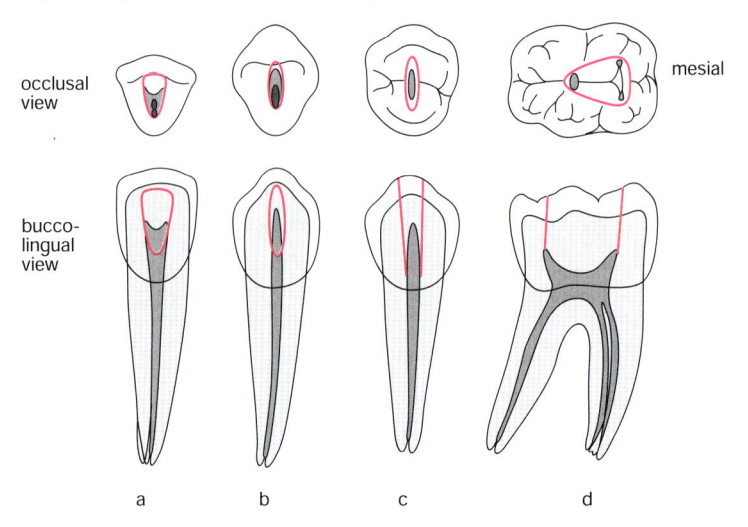

(a) Mandibular incisor. (b) Mandibular canine. (c) Mandibular premolar. (d) Mandibular molar.

Mandibular molars (Fig 4-8d)
Typical length: 21mm
Number of canals 3: mesial usually 2; distal usually 1.
Basic access outline: triangular, with apex just distal to mid-line.
Note that the distal canal emerges into the chamber from the distal. Straight-line entry is simple from the mesial and requires no extension of the cavity much beyond the centre of the occlusal surface. If the distal canal seems off-centre, there is probably a second canal, and the cavity should be widened buccolingually to form a rectangular outline.

The commonest error is to provide a poor flight-path to the mesial canals, with resultant instrument flexion and ledging (Fig 4-2).

Third-dimension curvatures should always be anticipated. Almost 40% of lower molars, for example, will have canals with greater curvature in the unseen bucco-lingual plane than the mesiodistal plane.

Entering the Canal System

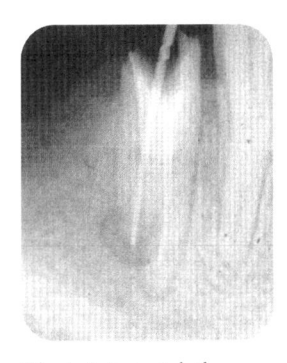

Fig 4-9 A straight bucco-lingual film during the initial treatment of this tooth left the second canal unidentified and untreated.

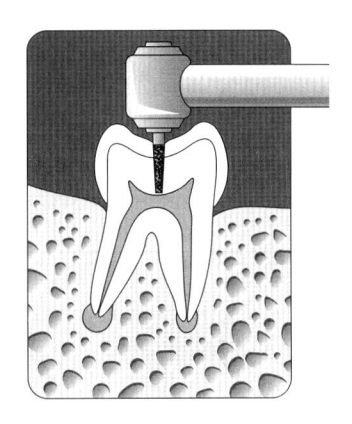

Fig 4-10 Routine orientation of line and length from an undistorted pre-operative film.

Radiographs

Preoperative radiographs should be life size, undistorted, well processed and, above all, inspected with care. It is often helpful to expose more than one film at different angles to build a three-dimensional picture of the tooth and the pulp system which formed it (Fig 4-9).

Quality preoperative radiographs provide information on:
- the depth and position of the chamber and its roof
- morphological changes which can make entry difficult (considered more fully in Chapter 5)
- orientation of depth and angulation (Fig 4-10).

Although coronal access is a relatively deep cavity, there is no merit in routinely choosing a long bur for the preparation. Why use a bur which can over-cut into a furca, when a shorter bur will reach the chamber and:
- be easier to accommodate with directional control in the vertical space available
- disallow further cutting before danger is reached?

Long-shanked burs should be reserved for cases in which they are needed.

Entering the Canal System

Fig 4-11 Practical stages of access.

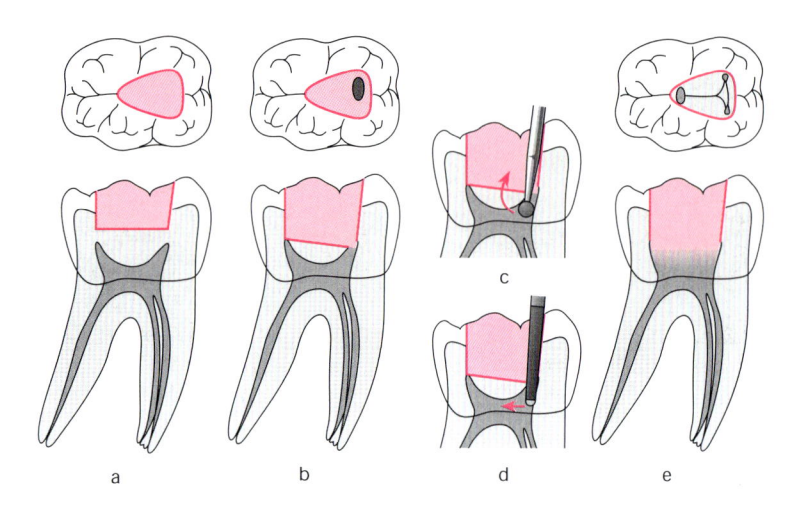

(a) Outlining the correct form, not simply stabbing in through a narrow, dark hole. (b) Initial puncture of the chamber roof. (c) Removing the roof with a slow-speed round bur, cutting on the outward stroke. (d) A safe-ended bur, directed around the walls of the chamber. The results are impressive and predictable. (e) An unroofed chamber.

Practical Stages

Outline and initial pulp access
If the tooth is sound or soundly restored, a classic outline is cut at high speed with a medium-tapered diamond bur (Fig 4-11a). As the cavity progresses, it is deepened in areas where the pulp is most prominent, and, at an anticipated depth, a satisfying drop may be felt as the bur falls through the roof (Fig 4-11b). Multiple punctures through the roof can be mistaken for canals (Fig 4-12a). Chamber floors are not flat and white, they are dark and domed with a map of lines guiding to canal entrances (Fig 4-12b).

The chamber can now be fully unroofed, either with:
- slow-speed round burs, cutting on the outward stroke (Fig 4-11c), or
- safe-ended access burs (Fig 4-13), introduced to the pulp exposure, and directed around the chamber walls to reveal its contents (Fig 4-11d, e).

These methods preserve the anatomy of the chamber floor and make life easier. If the floor is flattened or preparation extends beyond the lateral limit of

Entering the Canal System

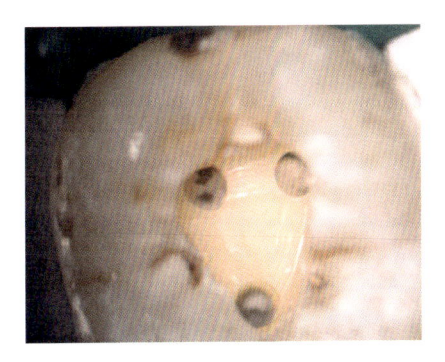

Fig 4-12a Multiple punctures through the chamber roof. Are these canals?

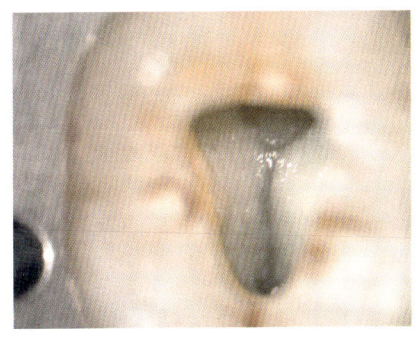

Fig 4-12b The unmistakable dark, domed and fissured chamber floor with its road map leading to canal entrances.

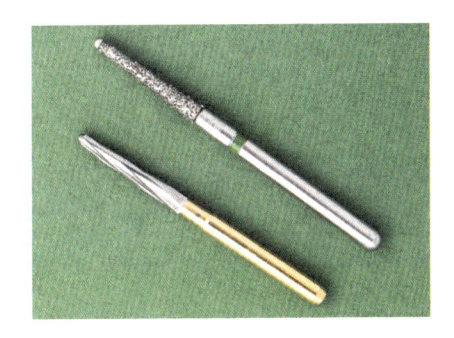

Fig 4-13 Safe-ended access burs: high-speed tungsten carbide Endo Z® and diamond Diamendo® (Maillefer/Dentsply).

the chamber, a helpful funnel is converted to an irritating flat surface with a small orifice (Fig 4-14). The result is a frustrating and time-wasting preparation in which the operator spends more time getting instruments into canals than using them when they are in. Safe-ended burs will stop that happening and transform the practice of most users.

Refinements
The chamber is now unroofed – but does it provide easy, straight-line access? A few moments should be spent considering the flight-paths of instruments, and making minor refinements for improvement. Many endodontists thought they made straight-line access until they started working with NiTi instruments which cannot be precurved. NiTi has forced a rethink of what we mean by straight-line access.

Entering the Canal System

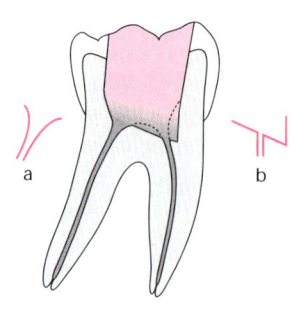

Fig 4-14 Time and frustration are saved by preserving the funnel-shaped entrances to canals **(a)**, rather than converting them to dots on flat surfaces **(b)**. Damage to this anatomy results in more time expended getting instruments into canals than using them for preparation when inserted.

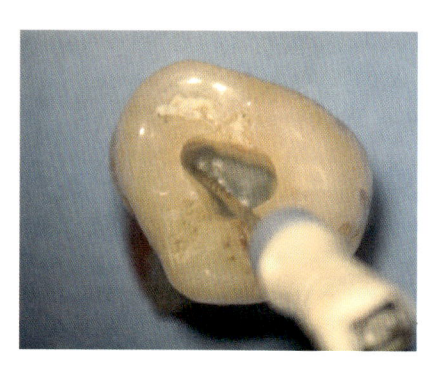

Fig 4-15a Access to an upper molar, but is the path to the mesiobuccal stress-free?

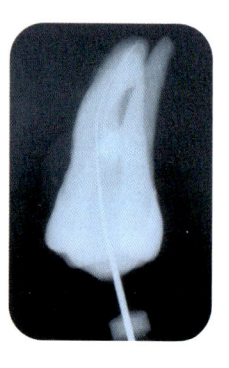

Fig 4-15b Radiographic image, showing instrument flexion.

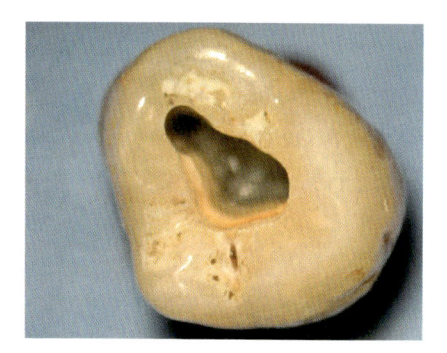

Fig 4-15c After countersinking the canal orifice, the wall was locally straightened to form a smooth chimney to the canal orifice.

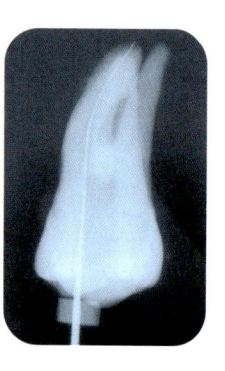

Fig 4-15d File entry is now less stressed, and instruments can be slid down the chimney rather than having to visualise the canal entrance; a great time and frustration-saver.

Entering the Canal System

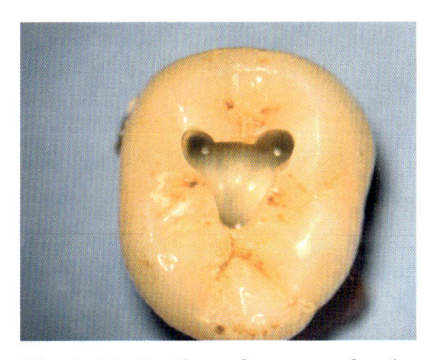

Fig 4-16 Similar refinements for the mesial canals of a lower molar.

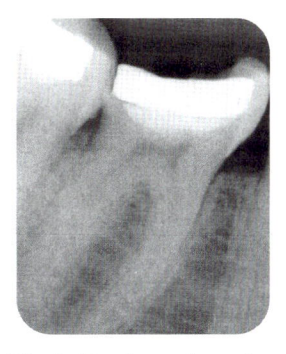

Fig 4-17a A simple molar to enter?

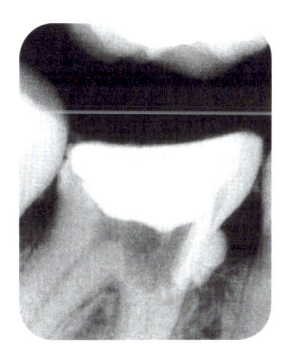

Fig 4-17b Correct orientation and the use of safe-ended burs should never have allowed this to happen.

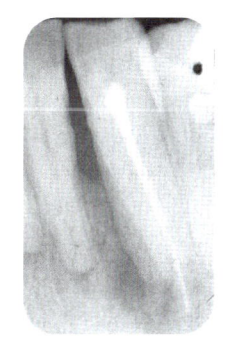

Fig 4-18 Failure by missing the anatomy through an under-prepared access.

Adequate access to an upper molar is shown in Fig 4-15a, but entry to the mesiobuccal canal is hardly straight (Fig 4-15b). By countersinking the canal entrance with a Gates-Glidden drill size 3, space is made to accommodate the tip of a safe-ended access bur which can locally straighten the path to the canal entrance by removing a bulging overhang of cervical dentine (Fig 4-15c,d). The junction may need to be blended-in with a Gates or hand file. For the investment of a few seconds and a small amount of tooth tissue, access is now straight and stress-free. Similar, rational cavity refinements are shown for the mesial canals of a lower molar in Fig 4-16.

The canal orifice no longer needs to be seen; instruments will glide to length down the smooth chimneys which have been formed.

The chamber should be flooded with sodium hypochlorite to stem bleeding from pulp stumps and start the process of disinfection and pulp digestion.

Common errors
Over-preparation usually results from loss of orientation and the use of inappropriate tools. Following the guidelines presented in this chapter, the molar shown in Fig 4-17a should have been accessed in minutes and with no fear of damage. Instead, it was perforated mesially and into the furca, and the mesial half of the tooth is now unrestorable (Fig 4-17b).

Under-preparation can be equally serious, with missed anatomy, intractable infection and discolouration amongst its consequences (Fig 4-18).

Conclusions

- Access lies at the foundation of successful root canal treatment. Time and care taken at this stage rewards practitioners at all subsequent stages.
- Safe practice involves orientation of depth and angulation, avoidance of long burs unless necessary, and the routine application of safe-ended access burs to unroof the chamber without damage.
- When basic outline is complete, the cavity should be fine-tuned for simplified and stress-free entry.
- There is great value in occasionally inspecting, sectioning and accessing extracted teeth on the benchtop.

Further Reading

Burns RC, Herbranson EJ. Tooth morphology and cavity preparation. In: Cohen S, Burns RC (Eds.) Pathways of the Pulp. 8th ed. St Louis: Mosby, 2002:173-229.

Walton RE. Access preparation and length determination. In: Walton RE, Torabinejad M (Eds.) Principles and Practice of Endodontics. 3rd ed. Philadelphia: Saunders, 2002:182-205.

Chapter 5
Entering "Calcified" Systems

Aim
To describe common age changes which complicate pulp access and introduce methods which may assist entry.

Outcome
After studying this chapter, the reader should have greater understanding of changes which complicate entry to the aged tooth, and be conversant with a variety of techniques which may assist orientation and entry.

The Frustration of the "Calcified" Pulp

Entry to canal systems can be difficult. Most dentists know the frustration of the "calcified" tooth (Fig 5-1), a common finding in heavily restored teeth in ageing populations. Regrettably, such teeth are not immune to apical periodontitis. Compromise, referral or extraction are often the only solutions in practice.

Pulp space diminishes by:
- reduction of pulp chamber and canal volume
- calcified deposition within the chamber and canals.

These changes can present alone or in combination.

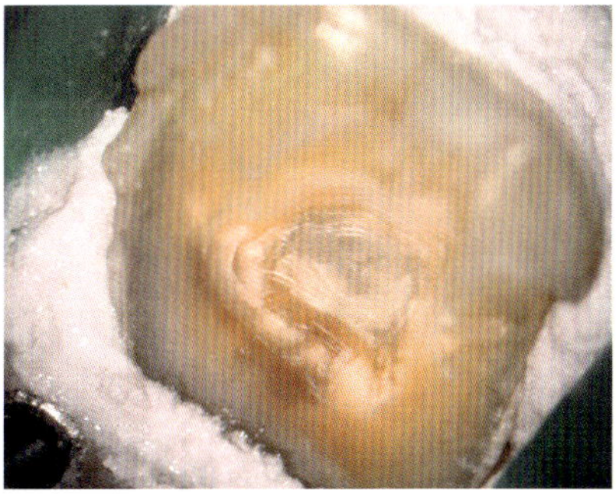

Fig 5-1 Facing a brick wall! The calcified pulp system of a middle-aged patient.

Entering "Calcified" Systems

Reduced Chamber and Canal Volume

Pulps continue to secrete dentine throughout life. In molars, this is mainly on the floor and roof of the chamber, converting it from a deep cavern to a flat disc (Fig 5-2a,b). This process also narrows the entrances and moves them closer to the centre of the tooth.
Incisor and canine pulps retreat out of the crown and centrally (Fig 5-2c,d).

The picture in the crown can be complicated by irregular "irritation" dentine, secreted to wall off tubules exposed by caries, dentistry and wear (Fig 5-3).

In roots, dentine deposition is always concentric. When searching and probing for the pulp in a root, it can only be in the centre of the mass of dentine which it formed (Fig 5-2b,d).

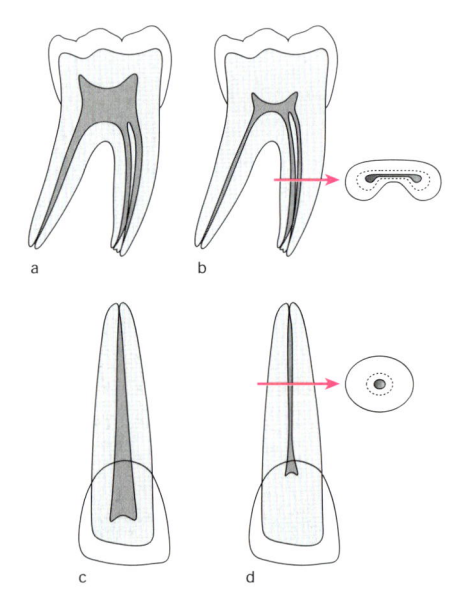

Fig 5-2 Age changes in pulp volume.

(a) Molar pulp system in a young adult. **(b)** Dentine deposition on the chamber roof and floor converts it to a flat disc which is easily traversed without realising by a poorly orientated bur. The first "give" can be the furca! The canal entrances also narrow and move centrally, whilst in cross-section, the canals narrow concentrically. **(c)** Incisor pulp system of a young adult. **(d)** Retreat of the coronal pulp apically and centrally. In cross-section, the root canal again narrows concentrically.

What About Apical Calcification?

Failure to reach length in a canal is often blamed on apical calcification. In truth, canals do not suddenly calcify in their apical reaches, and are more commonly wider in this protected apical region than further coronally where external irritants can provoke dentine deposition. Deep obstructions usually represent:
- impacted debris
- compacted pulp tissue
- abrupt canal curvatures, often in a plane which is not visible in normal radiographic views.

The illusion of apical calcification can also arise as tapered instruments are advanced into canals with parallel or coronally narrowed walls (Fig 5-4). The interference actually lies coronally, causing the instrument to hang-up, making apical progress difficult, and rationalised in the mind of the operator as an apical blockage.

Calcified Inclusions

Islands of calcification form around degenerating blood vessels and nerve fibres in the pulp. These glassy translucent deposits are not strictly dentine, and can appear very dense on radiographs. In the coronal pulp, they are usually spheroidal "pulp stones" (Fig 5-8), interspersed with fronds of soft tissue which provide cleavage-planes for disruption and removal. Some may become firmly attached by incorporation into secondary dentine deposits on the chamber floor or walls.

Pulp stones are replaced in root canals by linear calcifications. Interspersed again with soft tissue, they have the texture of a wet cocktail stick and will cause a sharp probe to stick. Only caries, canal entrances and linear deposits will stick on probing – a helpful strategy in identifying and developing canals for entry.

Fig 5-3 Irregular, irritation dentine laid down to wall-off tubules opened by caries.

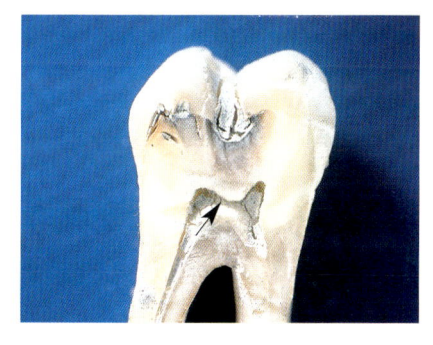

Entering "Calcified" Systems

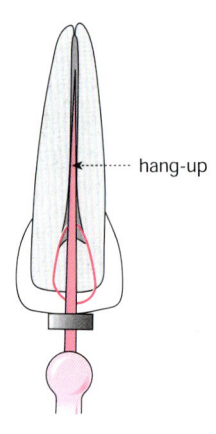

Fig 5-4 Hang-up of a file giving the illusion of apical obstruction. Opening the canal coronally allows the file to drop deeper.

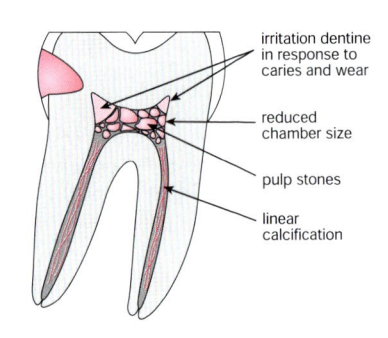

Fig 5-5 The composite aged tooth, with diminution of pulp volume by regular and irritation dentine deposition, and obliteration of this space with pulp stones coronally and linear deposits in the roots.

The apparent density of calcified inclusions on radiographs belies their soft tissue component, which harbours the microorganisms responsible for apical periodontitis, whilst greatly assisting entry.

The composite aged tooth is illustrated in Fig 5-5.

Entering the "Calcified" Chamber

Vision and orientation are critical:
- good light
- a front-silvered mirror
- magnification

are indispensable aids. In an ideal world, all would have the use of an operating microscope, but even the simplest of loupes will provide an edge.
Guidelines for depth orientation and bur selection were presented in Chapter 4.
Depth and direction of cut should be constantly reviewed and small bleeding points checked with an electronic apex locator before they are assumed to be pulp exposures and opened widely (Fig 5-6). If a perforation is identified, bleeding should be controlled with sodium hypochlorite and paper

Entering "Calcified" Systems

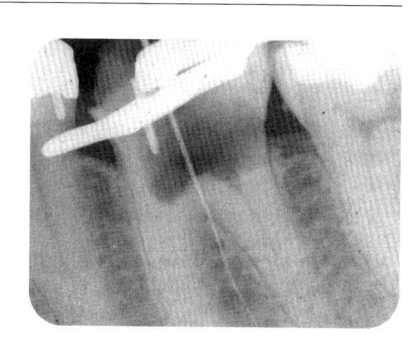

Fig 5-6 Check the identity of bleeding spots before opening them widely. Perforations should be dried and sealed immediately.

points, before making an immediate repair with an adhesive material or Mineral Trioxide Aggregate (Maillefer/Dentsply).

Safe-ended access burs again allow safe removal of the chamber roof to its lateral limits, though progress may not be rapid if the chamber is shallow or filled with pulp stones.

Removing Pulp Stones

Pulp stones can usually be disrupted and removed along cleavage planes. A sharp spoon excavator or probe may be sufficient, but an ultrasonic scaler is especially useful and friendly to the chamber floor. If a bur is needed, it should be one with a narrow shank such as a:
- goose-neck® (Meissinger)
- long-neck (LN)® bur (Maillefer/Dentsply) (Fig 5-7).

The aim is to pick up the dark, domed floor of the chamber and find its fissured road-map which will lead to the canal orifices. It is wise to remove any loose calcified material from the chamber to avoid the risk and frustration of it falling into canals and blocking them (Fig 5-8).

Entering Canals With Linear Deposits

There should be no urgent hurry to pick up files. Unless there is a clear path for them to follow, they will repeatedly bend and quickly form an expensive pile of casualties. Possible entrances should be explored first with a long DG16 canal probe, inserted with firm pressure to detect a sticking point. If the probe does not stick, there is no path for a file to follow and excavation should continue with a goose-neck® or LN® bur, constantly checking orientation and probing. This process continues until:

Entering "Calcified" Systems

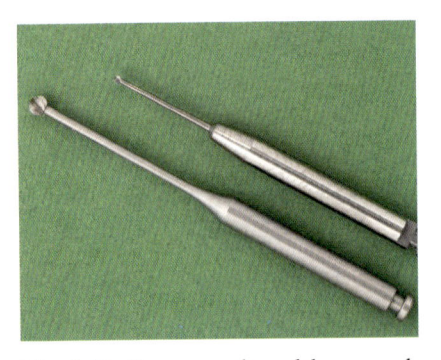

Fig 5-7 Goose-neck and long-neck (LN) pin burs for unroofing chambers and chasing canals. The narrow shaft allows the working head to be watched at all times.

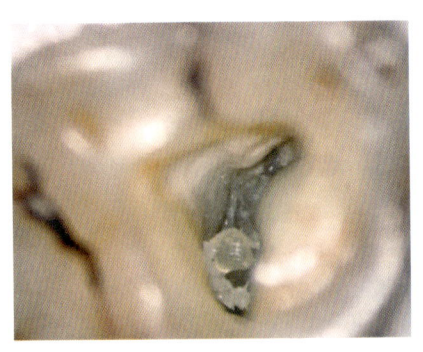

Fig 5-8 Work underway to unroof the road map in a molar.

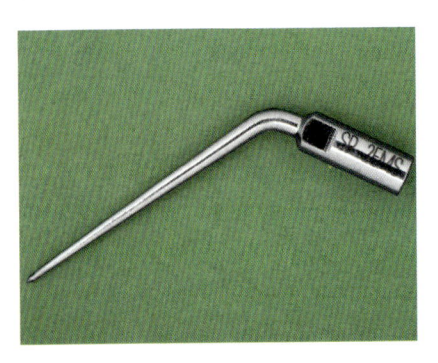

Fig 5-9 Cutting tip powered by ultrasound.

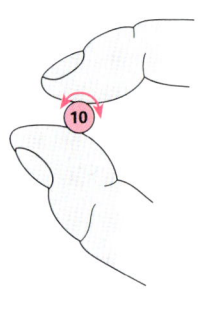

Fig 5-10 Watch-winding walks a small file into the canal. If the instrument feels tight, gently pull to remove dentine, free the instrument and allow the entry of more lubricant.

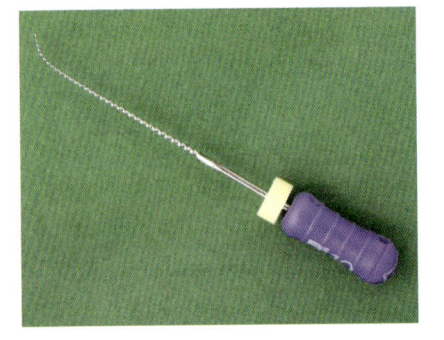

Fig 5-11 Small file smoothly curved in its apical 2-3mm to negotiate an apical curve. Directional rubber stops can be helpful.

- common sense suggests stopping or
- a convincing stick is felt.

Only then should small files be introduced.

Careful dentine removal can also be achieved with fine, cutting tips attached to a piezoelectric ultrasonic unit (Fig 5-9). However, control can be difficult without magnification and it is easy to burn the dentine and obscure landmarks.

Walking In

Files, size 10 or lower, should now be inserted with lubrication. The action of the file is a "watch wind": twiddling the instrument back and forth between forefinger and thumb pad with little or no vertical pressure (Fig 5-10). The file should walk its way into the canal. If progress is tight, twiddling will only lock the instrument tighter. The file should be pulled back to free it and "pick" debris away before proceeding. Twiddling and picking, the file will often reach a point where it suddenly drops into the wider apical portion of the canal and progress becomes simpler.

It is unclear whether the role of proprietary EDTA-containing gels is simply to ease the glide-path of instruments or to soften dentine. Whichever is true, instruments enter more easily with such agents or even with liquid medicated soap.

Tight or Loose Resistance?

If progress remains difficult, note should be made of how the instrument feels. If there is a slight sticking sensation as the file is withdrawn, this is tight resistance; the file is probably following the canal. Progress should continue, watch-winding and picking until the root terminus is reached or no further progress is possible.

If the instrument is loose in the canal but is making no further progress, the canal is probably curving, often in an unseen third dimension. The apical 2-3mm of a small file should be smoothly curved (Fig 5-11) and walked around all walls of the canal in an effort to find a stick spot which can be chased. Many files carry directional stops which assist file orientation deep in the canal. It should be remembered that the path which is sought does not necessarily lie at the depth of the preparation; it often exits on the lateral wall of the hole which has been created.

Not all cases will be won to ideal length, but patient and systematic instrumentation will allow entry to most systems for effective infection control.

Obstructing Non-calcified Canals

Even the most simple of canals can be blocked during entry. Compacted pulp tissue can form as impassable a barrier as any calcification and is best avoided by gross pulp removal with barbed broaches.

In all cases, canal negotiation should be accompanied by lubrication with soap or a proprietary EDTA paste to help instruments glide into masses of tissue rather than simply compact them.

Subsequent blockages with dentine mud should be avoided by frequent, deep irrigation and occasional passage of a small (size 10 or lower) file through the full length of the canal, extending passively 1mm or so through the apical foramen to keep the entire canal patent and under control.

The chamber should always be flooded brim-full with sodium hypochlorite solution in preparation for formal cleaning and shaping.

Conclusions

- Calcified canal systems are increasingly common and can thwart conventional approaches to access.
- Age changes include both diminution of pulp volume and obliteration with calcified inclusions.
- Canal systems are rarely completely calcified.
- Light, magnification and patience are indispensable aids during the careful use of ultrasound, long burs and canal probes. Files should not be picked up until there is a path for them to follow.
- Compacted pulp tissue can provide as impassable an obstruction as calcified material.

Further Reading

Lovdahl PE, Gutmann JL. Problems in locating and negotiating fine and calcified canals. In: Gutmann JL, Dumsha TC, Lovdahl PE, Hovland EJ (Eds.) Problem Solving in Endodontics. 3rd ed. St Louis: Mosby, 1997:69-89.

Walton RE. Geriatric endodontics. In: Walton RE, Torabinejad M (Eds.) Principles and Practice of Endodontics. 3rd ed. Philadelphia: Saunders, 2002:545-560.

Chapter 6
Creating the Conditions for Periapical Health

Aims

To provide a comprehensive overview of the fundamental principles of root canal preparation in terms of infection control and creating an environment compatible with periapical health. To describe a variety of manual and mechanised methods of shaping canals for effective cleaning and sealing.

Outcome

After studying this chapter, the reader should understand: the role of mechanical enlargement, irrigation and medication in cleaning root canal systems; the shortcomings of traditional enlarging tools and action; and the advantages of contemporary file design, metallurgy and motion.

Principles of Preparation

Canal preparation is the key infection-controlling step. It secures periapical health by:
- cleaning the canal system to remove microorganisms, microbial toxin and substrate
- shaping to create an internal form which can be sealed throughout its length against microbial entry, nutrition and multiplication.

Cleaning and shaping occur simultaneously by the synergistic action of instruments, irrigants and local medicaments, the emphasis of which will vary according to the case. A wide, tapered canal in a tooth without apical periodontitis may, for example, require less mechanical shaping and disinfection than a fine canal in a tooth with apical periodontitis.

The Role of Enlarging Tools, Irrigants and Local Medicaments

Instruments enlarge canals by cutting dentine and provide:
- mechanical cleaning
- access for irrigation
- adequate shape for compaction of the root filling.

Creating the Conditions for Periapical Health

The best outcome from mechanical instrumentation is concentric enlargement of all major canals (Fig 6-1a). An ideal system would achieve this:
- safely
- predictably
- according to the cleaning needs of the canal, not to an empirical norm or a point dictated by instrument limitations.

Viewed longitudinally, it would always produce a smoothly tapering preparation with its narrowest point apically and its widest point coronally - currently the optimal shape for effective sealing (Fig 6-1b).

Irrigants support enlargement by lubricating the path of instruments and flushing cutting debris, which may otherwise cause blockages and compromise cleaning. Critically, they also clean the complex webs, fins, anastomoses and accessory canals which instruments will never be guided to enter (Fig 6-2). As such, they should have antimicrobial, and pulp-dissolving activity.

- Sodium hypochlorite solution remains the gold standard, usually thin household bleach (always protect the patient's eyes and clothes), diluted with an equal volume of water to give an approximately 2% solution. Greater or lesser dilution is also acceptable, though its cleaning activity increases with:
  - concentration
  - volume
  - temperature
  - agitation.
- Chlorhexidine gluconate (0.2%) is an acceptable alternative, with substantive antimicrobial action but no tissue-dissolving capacity.

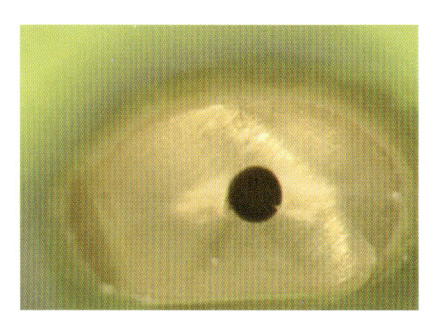

Fig 6-1a Concentrically enlarged root canal.

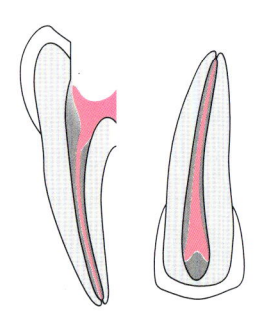

Fig 6-1b Longitudinally, preparations should be centred on the original canal and form smooth, regular tapers, from apical to coronal.

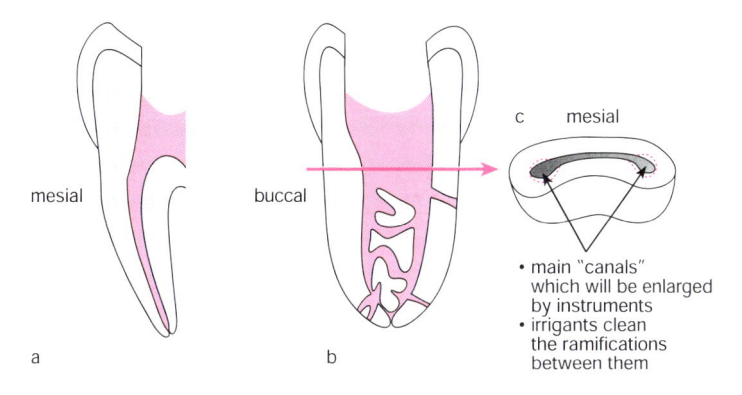

Fig 6-2(a) Typical mind's-eye view of a lower molar root canal in clinical, buccolingual view. **(b)** Closer to reality. Mesiodistal view of a lower molar mesial root, with areas of expansion "canals" buccally and lingually, curving in three dimensions, and with complex branching and interconnection at every level. **(c)** Cross-sectional view illustrating the web of communication between "canals". Enlarging instruments will shape the main canal areas, leaving the ramifications to be cleaned and disinfected with bleach.

- EDTA fluid or gel can be alternated to remove smear layer and open dentinal tubules for disinfection, though the merits of this action remain contentious.
- Local anaesthetic, the most popular irrigant, has neither antimicrobial nor tissue solvent activity and is an expensive agent to flush cutting debris.

Delivery is with narrow, safe-ended irrigating needles (Fig 6-3) which facilitate:
- deep
- high volume
- low pressure exchange.

They should be securely attached to a labelled Luer-Loc syringe. The plunger is depressed with a finger to limit pressure which could force solution beyond the apex. An added precaution is to fit a rubber stop or to bend the fine needle to allow depth orientation and prevent over-extension.

Frequent flushing refreshes the chemical activity of the irrigant and helps dislodge loose debris. The application of ultrasound to a flooded canal goes further by warming the solution and creating violent turbulence to scrub canal walls and ramifications. Ultrasonically activated sodium hypochlorite is probably the most effective cleaning regime in endodontics.

Local medicaments supplement instruments and irrigants and offer longer-

term inter-appointment cleansing. Traditional volatile agents such as paramonochlorophenol, whose vapours allegedly fumigate canal systems, are irritant and lose their antimicrobial effectiveness (but not their smell) within hours. Worthwhile alternatives include:
- non-setting calcium hydroxide, with its
  - high pH,
  - lasting, broad-spectrum antimicrobial activity and
  - ability to assist in dissolving necrotic pulp tissue.
- chlorhexidine gel (2%), with its lasting broad-spectrum antimicrobial action (including activity against *E. faecalis*).

Antibiotic drugs cannot be recommended and should be avoided when a disinfectant will do a similar or better job without the risk of selecting microbial resistance.

The Trials of Traditional Preparation

Canals have traditionally been enlarged with modestly tapered stainless steel instruments (Fig 6-4). After determining length, the apex was empirically

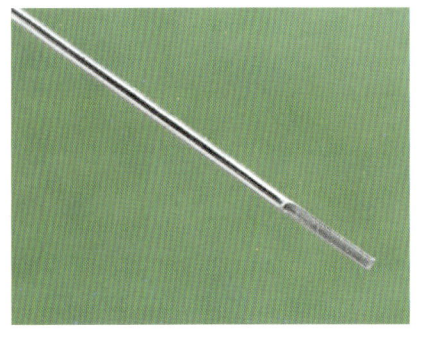

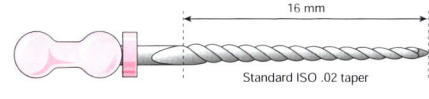

Fig 6-3 Safe-ended Monoject endodontic irrigating needle incorporating a cut-out area which guards against dangerous build-up of pressure and apical extrusion of canal contents. They should always be attached to a labelled Luer-Loc, not friction-grip syringe, and can be smoothly bent for depth orientation.

Fig 6-4 An ISO standardised endodontic file with 16mm of cutting blades and a standard, modest taper of 0.02mm mm^{-1}. For every mm of the bladed area, the instrument becomes 0.02mm wider. This standard was probably based on limitations of instrument manufacture in the middle of the last century rather than rationality of cleaning and shaping needs.

enlarged, before stepping back to create flare for filling. Instrument design and motion made for complex, time-consuming preparation, with limitless opportunity for error. Blockage and deviation of instruments from a centred position (transportation) were the norm.

Blockage resulted from:
- up-down filing motions which dislodged and packed debris
- preparation from apex to crown, instead of clearing debris as the case advanced in a crown-down sequence
- failure to check the free-running patency of the canal at frequent intervals during treatment.

The outcome was incompletely cleaned and filled canals.

Transportation resulted from:
- inflexible instruments, which straightened as they passed into curves, cutting on the outer wall apically and the inner wall coronally (Fig 6-5a)
- aggressive cutting tips which offered no restraint to file movement from a centred position
- repeated up-down filing motions. In curved roots, the canal, not the operator controls the instrument's position. Recurring up-down filing motions cause the instruments to cut repeatedly in the same place, forming an ever-deepening groove as they migrate from a centred position (Fig 6-5a,b).

This has been a daily reality in practice: ledged and inadequately cleaned canals, inadequately shaped for an effective seal.

Problems were compounded by the realisation that apical canal diameters remain large into old age and that rational enlargement for effective mechanical cleaning may be far greater than possible with traditional tools and motion.

Combating Transportation

Attempts to control transport have included:
- Anticurvature filing. This popular action, in which some walls were filed more than others, failed to recognise three-dimensional anatomy and the reality that the position of a file deep in a curved canal cannot be controlled by the earnest efforts of the dentist at the canal entrance.
- Pre-curving instruments to match radiographic canal curvatures. This two-dimensional solution again denied the unseen, often more severe buccolingual curvature and could not combat transportation.

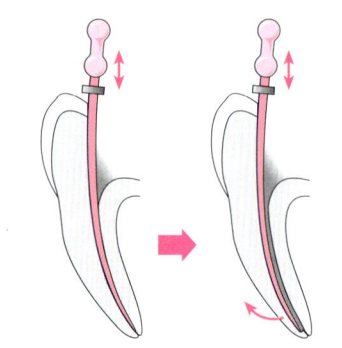

Creating the Conditions for Periapical Health

Fig 6-5 (a) Deviation of instruments from a long-axis centred position.

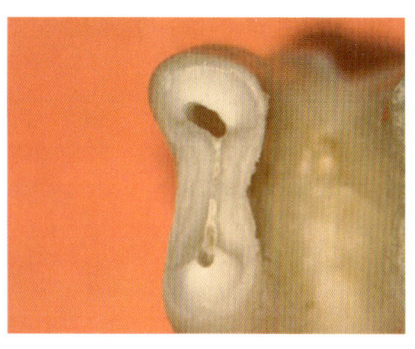

Fig 6-5 (b) The consequences of inflexible instruments being guided by canal curvature to cut repeatedly in the same place. The instrument in the upper canal transported from a centred position and loses shape. The lower canal was prepared bigger by rotation and remains centred.

- Limiting the extent of apical enlargement so that only small instruments reached the root terminus. This strategy disregarded apical canal diameter and the need to open for mechanical cleaning and irrigation. Sadly, even size 25 stainless steel files will transport curved canals when applied in a traditional filing motion, leaving them irregularly shaped and undercleaned. For reference, a narrow, 27 gauge irrigating needle equates to instrument size 45.

More recent and rational strategies have included:
- changes in file-tip geometry
- rotational, including Balanced-Force instrument motion
- more flexible metal alloys.

File-tip Geometry

Most endodontic files now have blunt tips and smooth angles of transition from the aggressive cutting area to the tip. Many also incorporate flat outer surfaces – "radial lands" (Fig 6-6) – which further restrict file movement from a central axis.

Rotational, Balanced-Force Cutting

A dramatic improvement in the safety and efficiency of K-file performance came with the description of Roane's Balanced-Force motion in 1985. Briefly, the file is gently inserted and rotated a quarter-turn clockwise to engage the blades in dentine (Fig 6-7a). If the file is turned further or harder, it may lock and twist-off during removal, leaving the tip *in situ*.

The cutting stroke involves anti-clockwise rotation. If the file is simply rotated anti-clockwise, it will screw out of the canal without cutting. In order to cut, it must be turned anti-clockwise, whilst pressing (Fig 6-7b) to balance the force with which it wants to back out. This will be smaller with a small file than a large one. As the file is held by vertical pressure and rotated, tension builds in its shank until the energy it contains balances and overcomes the force with which it is being held in dentine. A click is heard and felt as the dentine shears; a truly disconcerting experience at first with every expectation that the instrument has fractured.

Cutting debris is removed by rotating a quarter-turn clockwise once again (Fig 6-7c) to pick up broken dentine which is carried out on the flutes. After wiping and inspection for any damage, the file can be re-inserted and if it now rotates freely, it has cut a circle and done all the work it can; a rational time to move on to the next instrument.

For those with no experience of Balanced-Force motion, it will transform manual instrumentation into a safe and efficient process, but it must be practised to avoid excessive force, and to overcome fear of the clicks. The prize is a centred, circular preparation with little risk of ledging and transport because:

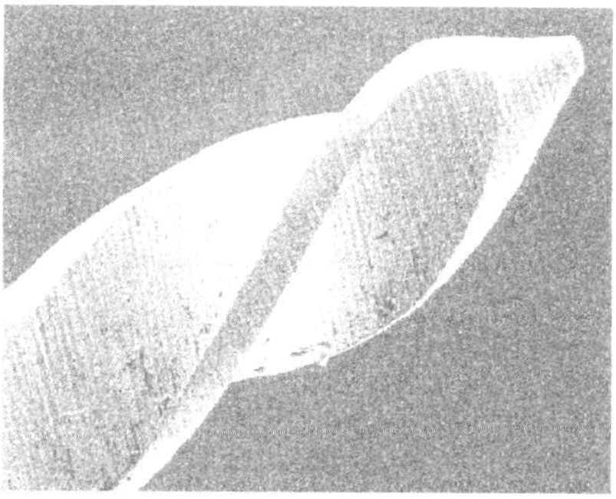

Fig 6-6 Non-end-cutting file with its rounded tip and smooth transition from bladed to non-bladed area. Radial lands at the periphery of many files also work to hold instruments centred in the canal.

Creating the Conditions for Periapical Health

Fig 6-7 The Balanced-Force motion.

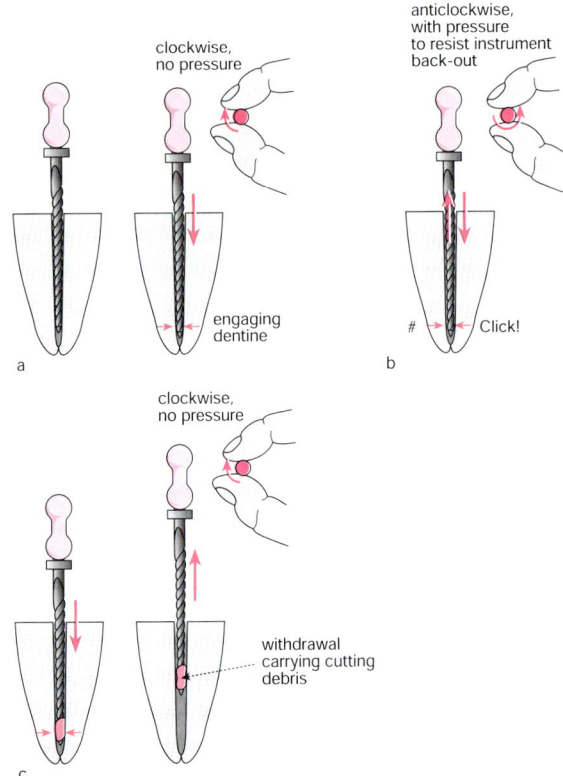

(a) Engaging dentine with a light quarter-clockwise turn. **(b)** The cutting stroke: turning anticlockwise safely screws the file out of the canal without cutting. This backing-out force must be balanced by pushing down on the instrument to prevent its retreat and cut dentine. There is a worrying click as the dentine shears. **(c)** Clearing cutting debris requires another light quarter-clockwise turn to pick up material on the flutes, and withdrawal to carry it free from the canal.

- instruments are not driving forward during the cutting phase, and
- repeated cutting strokes are avoided.

Flexible Metal Alloys

Metallurgy has brought other developments, first with more flexible stainless steel, then with nickel-titanium (NiTi) alloys. NiTi was introduced to endodontics in the late 1980s with the benefits of:

- unprecedented flexibility
- the ability to be milled into a variety of conventional and radical new forms
- the ability to withstand repeated flexion (cyclic fatigue/work hardening), and rotate in curved canals with reduced risk of fracture.

NiTi has opened an exciting age of mechanical root canal preparation, with consistent, well-centred preparations achievable by hand, or with engine-driven assistance.

Flexible instruments with greatly increased tapers mill smooth, predetermined tapers by default, without the need for complex step back procedures, and apical preparations can be matched to the diameter and cleaning needs of the canal, not the flexibility limits of enlarging tools. Properly trained novices as well as experienced dentists have been empowered.

Other Advances in Canal Preparation

Improvements in instrument manufacture and action have not been the only changes to simplify and rationalise canal preparation.

Early Flaring/Crown-down Preparation

Most techniques now open the coronal third of the canal before working deeper, and many prepare entirely from crown to apex for the following reasons:
- Most of the infected, necrotic material lies in the coronal half of the canal. By eliminating this material early, it is less likely to be carried apically during subsequent preparation, reducing the incidence of blockage and post-operative flare-up.
- Irrigant solutions do not exchange far beyond the tip of the delivery needle. Early flaring or progressive crown-to-apex preparation allows deep entry at an early stage, reducing the risk of blockage and potentiating cleaning.
- Difficult advance of a small instrument is usually rationalised as "apical sclerosis". The reality is often "hang-up" in the coronal third of the canal, and early flaring frees deeper entry (Fig 5-4).

A crown-down approach also commends that apical instrumentation is the finale, allowing sensitive, interference-free sizing and rational enlargement of this critical region.

Maintaining Patency

Canals are still easy to block if checks are not made frequently and steps taken to free them before they become firmly established.

It has become common practice to advance a small file up to, or even 1mm through, the apical foramen at intervals during preparation to ensure that length is maintained. This action remains controversial, but the dangers of an infected apical plug probably outweigh those of a small instrument (size 10 or lower) occasionally passing through the apical constriction without enlargement. This is not licence to blunder long with larger instruments.

Maintenance of canal patency actually allows preparation to proceed in any sequence desired and gives the option to advance the length of instrumentation at any stage if the need arises.

Electronic Length Determination

The optimal place to end canal preparation is where inside becomes outside; the cemento-dentinal junction, or "apical constriction" (Fig 6-8). This is said to lie between 0.5 and 2mm short of root end: a very imprecise guideline for practice.
The majority of dentists use radiographs and measured instruments for length determination, and it is likely that inadvertent under- or over-preparation occurs routinely. More accurate length determination can be achieved with contemporary electronic apex locators which have proved themselves in

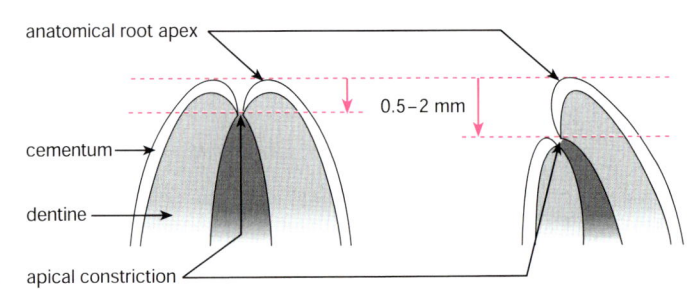

Fig 6-8 The apical constriction, physiological apex or cemento-dentine junction, where inside (inaccessible to host defences) becomes outside (accessible to host defences) – the optimal place to end preparation.

clinical research and experience. Current devices are accurate in wet and dry canals (Table 6-1).

For all their accuracy, apex locators can only convey information on length, not the range of diagnostic information available from a good-quality film. They may rationalise and streamline the use of radiographs but they should not do away with them completely.

Good-quality mid-treatment films can be secured with a dedicated film holder (Fig 6-9), separating individual roots by exposing at a slight off-angle.

Getting Ready for Preparation

Lubrication, gross tissue removal and negotiation to length were discussed in Chapter 5.

Regardless of the preparation technique to be used, it is helpful to do some initial opening by quickly running through standard K-files size 15-35, inserted passively, and rotated anticlockwise before withdrawal. The opened canal is then irrigated, and checked for patency as definitive preparation begins.

Techniques for Canal Preparation

In the following paragraphs, some contemporary methods will be reviewed for:
- manual preparation with ISO instruments
- manual preparation with increased taper instruments
- engine-driven (rotary) preparation with tapered and taperless instruments.

Table 6-1 **Some electronic apex locators which perform well in wet and dry canals.**

Apit (Osada)
Apex Finder AFA (Analytic)
Justy II (Panadent)
Raypex 4 (VDW)
Root ZX (Morita)

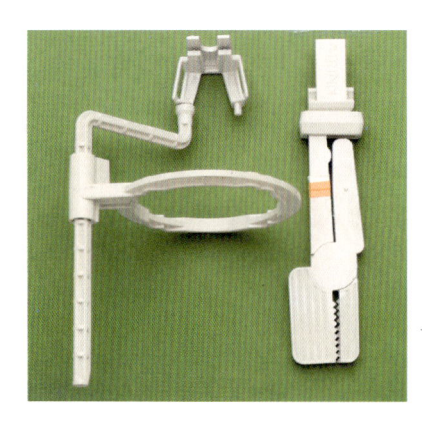

Fig 6-9 Rinn Endo-Ray and Snap-a-Ray film holders for undistorted mid-treatment images.

Manual Preparation with ISO Instruments

ISO instruments still have a place, and "stepdown", "double flare" or variants of these techniques with ISO files remain standard teaching in most undergraduate programmes (Fig 6-10).

Coronal flaring
- After access, exploration and initial passive opening with K-files, the straight, coronal half to two-thirds of the canal is opened with Gates Glidden drills 2, 3 and 4, inserted without force and directed lightly against canal walls on withdrawal. In multi-rooted teeth, they are directed away from furcal walls which are at risk of over-thinning and perforation (Fig 6-10a,b). Increasing sizes are inserted to shallower depths, and the canals irrigated and checked for patency.

Working length determination
- This can be achieved electrically, radiographically or by a combination of methods. The advantage of determining working length after coronal flaring is that the distance from apical constriction to coronal reference point is less likely to alter. If coronal flaring happens after working length determination, the distance from apical constriction to coronal reference point shortens. Studiously measuring instruments to the previously determined working length, the canal is inadvertently prepared long, with no apical stop and a dissatisfying overfill.

Initial apical enlargement
- The canal is now prepared to working length with gentle Balanced-Force motions. There is no possibility of gauging canal diameter at this stage of

Creating the Conditions for Periapical Health

Fig 6-10 Stepdown or Double-Flare preparation with standard ISO instruments.

(a) Flaring the straight, coronal part of the canal (first flare) with Gates Glidden drills. Increasing sizes are inserted to lesser depths, and all are directed away from furcal walls to prevent over-thinning. **(b)** Over-thinning and near strip-perforation from careless enlargement. **(c)** Initial apical enlargement to arbitrary size 25 opens the apical region for irrigant exchange, but definitive preparation must wait until the canal is properly flared. **(d)** Flaring the apical part of the canal (second or double flare) to blend smoothly with the coronal area. This can be achieved by stepping back from the apex in 1mm increments or enlarging from coronal to apical. **(e)** Revision of the apical preparation as the finale. Files act as feeler gauges of canal diameter, making apical preparation rational.

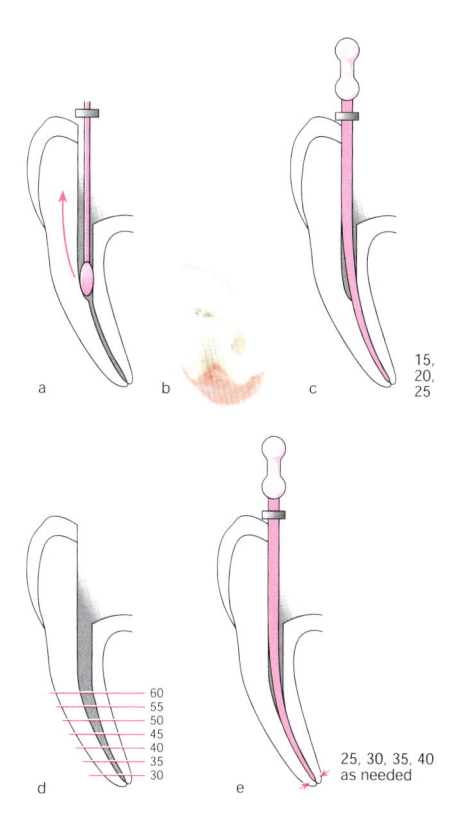

the preparation, and the apical region is opened initially to an arbitrary size 25 (Fig 6-10c). With Balanced-Force motion, this is small enough to avoid serious transport in all but the most severely curved canals.

Flaring for deep shape
- The canal is now flared with larger K-files, stepping back with Balanced-Force motion to size 60 at 0.5-1mm intervals (Fig 6-10d). Step back occurs rapidly and a freely rotating instrument marks rational progress to the next instrument which is accompanied by irrigation and patency checks.
- There is no reason why this flaring cannot be developed crown-down, starting where the Gates 2 reached with a size 60 file and working progressively apically.

71

Creating the Conditions for Periapical Health

Apical gauging and revision
- The canal properly flared, there is now an opportunity to gauge apical canal diameter. This phase is best completed with flexible NiTi files which will allow the canal to be enlarged for its cleaning needs without the constraints imposed by inflexibility (Fig 6-10e).

- The size 25 file is inserted, and usually passes to length without resistance. This is often surprisingly followed by size 30 and 35 instruments which loosely sweep to length. This process of apical gauging continues until resistance is felt, and Balanced-Force motion cuts dentine in the apical 1-2mm. In addition to the clicking, cutting sensation, cut dentine will be visible on the tip of the file as it is withdrawn (Fig 6-11). Rational apical enlargement.

Molar root canals are often prepared to size 40 by this method, and have clean apices with good resistance form for obturation.

Final checks
- A radiographic or electronic check with master files in place can be helpful to finalise preparation.
- All condensing instruments should then be tried in the canal to ensure that they will be able to pack the root filling throughout its length.

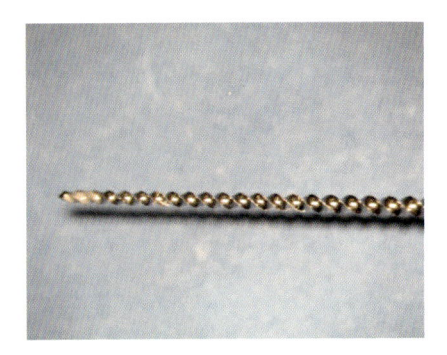

Fig 6-11 Flute-loading during apical revision. Apical diameter is known because it is clear when dentine has been cut; cleaning is improved and master cone fit is predictable.

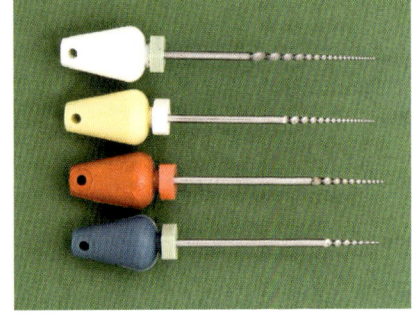

Fig 6-12 GT hand files with common, size 20 tips, maximum bladed diameter of 1mm, oversize pear-shaped handles and blades milled in reverse for clockwise Balanced-Force motion.

Manual Preparation with Increased-taper Instruments

Manual preparation is simpler and more consistent with NiTi Greater Taper hand files (GT files: Maillefer/Dentsply).
These have:
- 3, 4, 5 or 6 times the standard file taper (Table 6-2) to deliver smooth, predictable preparations
- size 20, non-cutting tips
- a maximum bladed diameter of 1mm (size 100), making the active region shorter as taper increases (Fig 6-12) to limit unhelpful file rigidity and excessive coronal dentine removal
- over-sized, pear-shaped handles for relatively high rotational cutting forces and to balance the strong outward force during rotation
- blades milled in reverse to deliver Balanced-Force motion by clockwise rotation.

Preparation is usually completed with one instrument, working from crown to apex to create a preparation of its own size and taper, the "final shaping objective". Root size and curvature dictate "final shaping objective" instrument selection (Table 6-2).

Table 6-2 **Greater Taper (GT) hand files and final shaping objectives.**

Handle colour	Taper	Final shaping objective
White	.06 (3 times ISO)	Mandibular incisors, 2 rooted premolars, other fine or severely curved canals
Yellow	.08 (4 times ISO)	Everything else
Red	.10 (5 times ISO)	
Blue	.12 (6 times ISO)	Maxillary central incisors, distal roots of mandibular molars, palatal roots of maxillary molars

Typical preparation

Initial entry
- Negotiation and passive opening is recommended, as previously.

Crown-down shaping
- Preparation follows with the final shaping objective file in clockwise Balanced-Force motion (Fig 6-13a). The instrument is removed frequently, wiped and inspected for faults and the canal irrigated and checked for patency.
- Working length is determined as the apical third is reached, and the preparation continued to the determined length.
- Alternatively, the .12, .10, .08 and .06 files can be used in crown-down sequence.

Apical gauging
- Standard NiTi instruments can then be inserted to working length to gauge canal diameter and revise the apical preparation, as previously.
- In canals which are narrow apically, passive insertion of files 20, 25, 30,

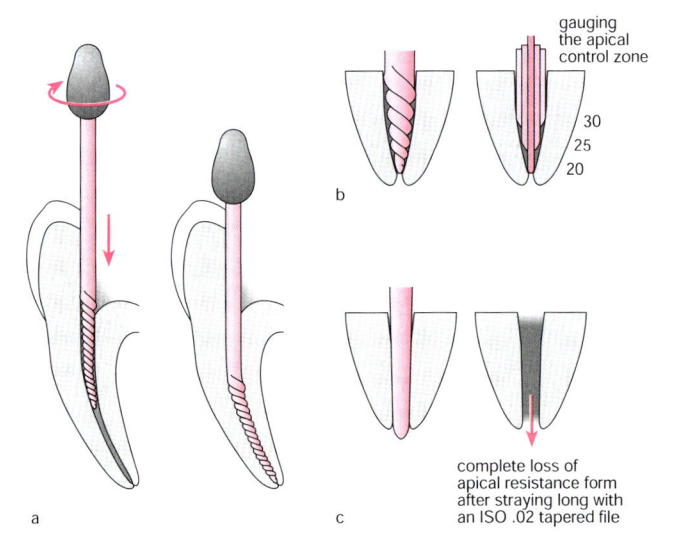

Fig 6-13(a) Crown-down preparation with the final shaping objective GT file. **(b)** Apical gauging of canal preparation and apical control zone. The apical control zone preserves apical resistance form even if the instrument is over-extended. **(c)** Loss of length control with an over-extended ISO tapered instrument.

35, 40 will confirm the development of smooth apical taper (Fig 6-13b). The apical preparation in this circumstance is not a traditional stop, but a rapidly tapering "apical control zone". The likely advantage is that if instrumentation was long, resistance to overfill has not been lost. By contrast, straying an ISO tapered instrument long in traditional preparation loses all resistance form (Fig 6-13c).

Engine-driven Preparation with Tapered and Taperless NiTi Instruments

Since their introduction in the early 1990s NiTi rotary instruments have become indispensable tools for canal enlargement.
Before reviewing systems in greater detail, some generalities should be noted.

What We All Need to Know about Rotary NiTi

- Access must be straight. There is no possibility to bend NiTi instruments for a favourable flightpath, and access must be properly defined and revised.
- They are not boring tools or pathfinders, they are reamers - instruments for enlarging an existing hole. Grinding a path into the unknown demands pressure, and may lead to abrupt tip bending or dangerous blundering into areas of complex anatomy, severe curvature or confluence; a recipe for instrument fracture. Canal systems should be thoroughly explored and passively opened before rotary enlargement.
- Speed and feed are critical. Speed of rotation should be known, consistent and in accordance with the manufacturer's instructions. This is best delivered with an electric motor and speed-reducing handpiece. Instruments should be running smoothly throughout their advance and withdrawal from the canal. Feed refers to the rate of advance of a cutting tool into the canal. NiTi instruments should nibble (not bite) dentine, and should be advanced with low-amplitude up-down pecking motions, applying no more force than with a sharp pencil. Heavy advance can lock and shear instruments. No tool should be in the canal for longer than five seconds before withdrawal for cleaning and inspection.
- Torque control motors can further minimise the risk of locking and overload, stopping forward rotation or even backing out if a tool is used close to its torsional limit.
- Instruments should be constantly moving. Although NiTi withstands cyclic fatigue, it is concentrated in one place if an instrument is held still. One rotation at a given level cuts a concentric circle - repeated entry or dwelling at length brings no benefit.

- Instruments must be tracked. Unlike stainless steel instruments, NiTi rotaries can show few signs of stress before fracture. Systems must be in place to log and discard tools which have been used in a specified number of cases (usually ten). Particularly challenging cases should be credited as "more than one use".
- If something feels "wrong", NiTi rotaries should be withdrawn and the canal re-established with conventional instruments.
- There is a learning curve. Reading a manual is not enough, and new NiTi users must:
  - undertake a hands-on course
  - practice with extracted teeth
  - start on easy cases.

A range of tapered and non-tapered rotary systems are available (Table 6-3).

Tapered NiTi Rotary Systems

All of these incorporate:
- instruments of increased taper
- crown-down preparation
- apical preparation as the finale.

Table 6-3 **A range of tapered and taperless NiTi rotary systems.**

Tapered	GT systems	GT files (Dentsply)
	.06 taper systems	K3 (Kerr)
		ProFile (Dentsply)
	642 systems	HERO 642 (MicroMega)
		Flexmaster (VDW)
	Progressive taper systems	ProTaper (Dentsply)
Taperless		Lightspeed (Lightspeed Technologies)

Creating the Conditions for Periapical Health

All involve:
- frequent, high-volume irrigation with sodium hypochlorite
- patency checks
- gel lubricants to cut down friction and ease instrument glide-paths.

1. **Rotary GT**

Developed from the hand GT system, rotary preparation is quicker and less physically demanding (Fig 6-14).

Typical preparation (Fig 6-15)
- Negotiate and passively open the canal.
- Enlarge the orifice with Gates Glidden drills or the .12 GT file running at 5,000 rpm (Fig 6-15a).
- Select the final shaping objective instrument and advance steadily (not pecking up and down) at 150rpm for not more than five seconds.
- Remove the instrument for cleaning and damage inspection, canal irrigation and patency check.
- Continue to progress apically until working length is reached (Fig 6-15b).
- Apical gauging is exactly as described for the manual GT preparation, but further rotary enlargement is possible with accessory files of tip size 35, 50 and 70.

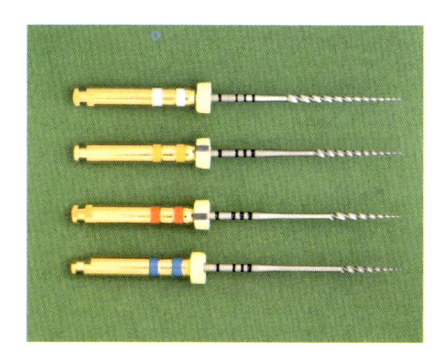

Fig 6-14 A standard set of four GT rotary files, sharing dimensions with hand-versions.

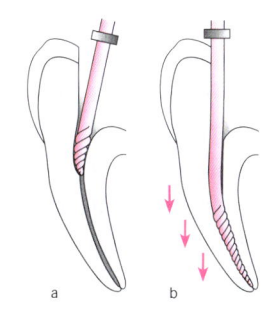

Fig 6-15 Typical GT rotary preparation. **(a)** Coronal flaring with the GT .12 taper file. **(b)** Preparation to root-end with the final shaping objective file. Again, all four instruments can be used in crown-down sequence if desired.

2. .06 tapered systems

Three times the ISO taper, a standard set contains instruments of tip size 40-15 (Fig 6-16), applied in a crown-down sequence at 150rpm.

Typical preparation (Fig 6-17)
- Negotiate and passively open the canal.
- Advance the size 40 instrument with gentle up-down pecking motions for no more than five seconds. Withdraw the instrument still running, wipe and inspect for damage.
- Irrigate the canal and check patency.
- Repeat with the size 35, 30, 25, 20 and 15 instruments until the apical 2mm is reached (Fig 6-17a).
- More than one passage through the series may be needed to reach this depth (Fig 6-17b), demanding patience and light touch.

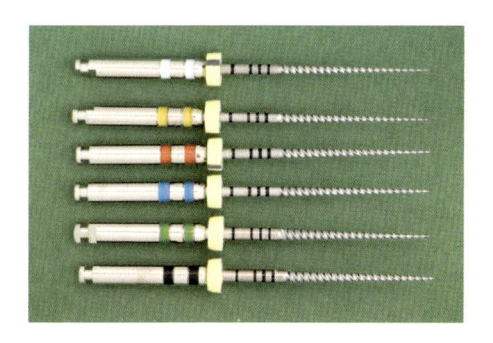

Fig 6-16 A standard set of .06 taper instruments, with three times the ISO taper and tip sizes 40-15.

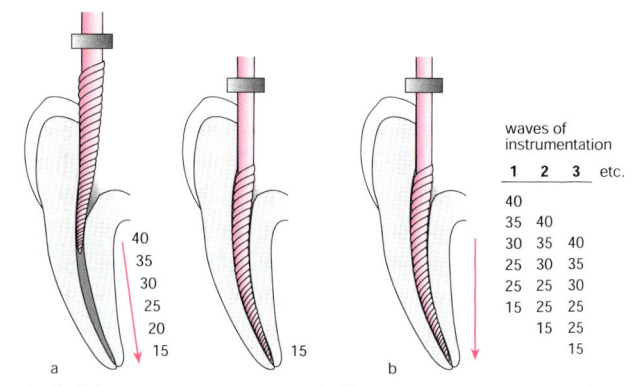

Fig 6-17 Typical .06 taper preparation. **(a)** Crown to apex preparation, starting with the size 40 instrument. **(b)** More than one passage through the series may be needed to reach working length.

Creating the Conditions for Periapical Health

- Apical diameter can then be gauged and enlarged to create a stop with standard NiTi hand files, or with .06 taper NiTi rotaries to create a fully .06 tapered preparation with an apical control zone.

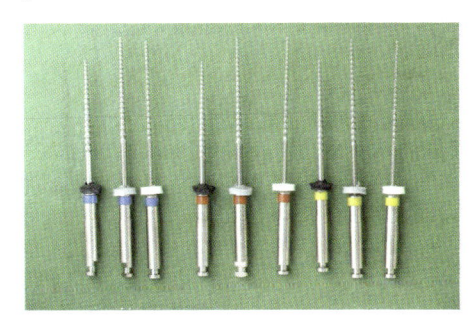

Fig. 6-18 642 systems with .06, .04 and .02 tapered instruments in a range of tip sizes.

3. 642 systems

Crown-down preparation is achieved by varying tip size and taper. A standard kit (Fig 6-18) contains .06, .04 and .02 tapered instruments in tip sizes 30-20. Generally, .06 tapers open the coronal half, .04 tapers shape to within 2mm of working length, and .02 tapers finish apically.

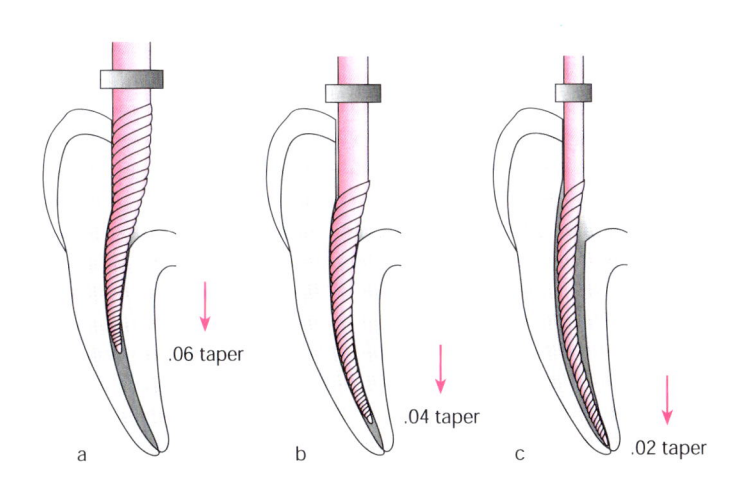

Fig 6-19 Typical 642 preparation. **(a)** .06 taper preparation for the coronal half to two-thirds of the canal. **(b)** .04 taper preparation to within 2mm of working length. **(c)** Apical gauging and stop preparation, either by hand or with .02 tapered rotaries.

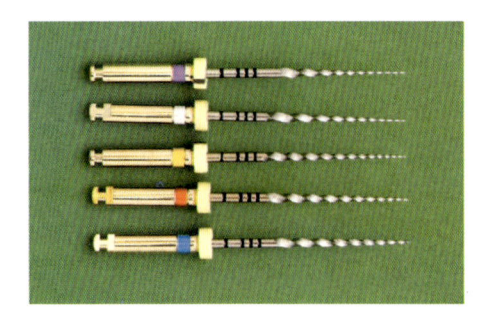

Creating the Conditions for Periapical Health

Fig. 6-20 Standard kit of progressively tapered instruments.

Table 6-4 **Standard kit of progressively tapered instruments and their dimensions.**

Instrument	Tip diameter	Maximum diameter	Taper
Shaper 1	.185mm (size 18.5)	1.19mm (size 119)	From .02 at tip to .11 at widest point
Shaper 2	.20mm (size 20)	1.19mm (size 119)	From .04 at tip to .115 at widest point
Finisher 1	.20mm (size 20)	1.13mm (size 113)	From .07 at tip to .05 at widest point
Finisher 2	.25mm (size 25)	1.2mm (size 120)	From .08 at tip to .05 at widest point
Finisher 3	.30mm (size 30)	1.2mm (size 120)	From .09 at tip to .05 at widest point

Typical preparation (Fig 6-19)
- Negotiate and passively open the canal.
- For a wide, straight canal, commence with the size 30 .06 taper, advancing with light pecking motions at 300-600rpm to enlarge the coronal half or two-thirds of the canal (Fig 6-19a).
- Irrigate and check for patency.
- Continue with the size 30 .04 taper to within 2mm of working length (Fig 6-19b).
- Apical gauging and stop preparation can be completed with NiTi hand instruments or .02 taper rotaries (Fig 6-19c).

In finer or more curved canals, preparation may commence with the size 25 or 20 series. The 642 systems offer considerable versatility in approaching canals of all configurations. Changing tip diameter and taper avoids any instrument doing too much work and becoming over-stressed as the case develops.

4. Progressively Tapered Systems

In addition to the fixed-taper systems, instruments are available which incorporate a range of tapers in their active region. A standard kit with details of instrument dimensions is shown in Table 6-4 and Fig 6-20.

Typical preparation (Fig 6-21)
- Negotiate and passively open the canal.
- Crown-down preparation begins with the Shaper 1, advancing with light in-out pecking motions for no more than five seconds (Fig 6-21a).
- Irrigate and check patency.
- Continue with the Shaper 1 and 2 until the apical 1-2mm are reached.
- Gauge the apical diameter with standard NiTi hand files (Fig 6-21b).
- According to the apical diameter, preparation is completed with the Finisher 1 (tip diameter size 20), 2 (tip diameter size 25) and 3 (tip diameter size 30) (Fig 6-21c).

Progressive tapers reduce the number of instruments compared with .06 and 642 systems and are claimed to optimise:
- light cutting
- flexibility
- fracture resistance.

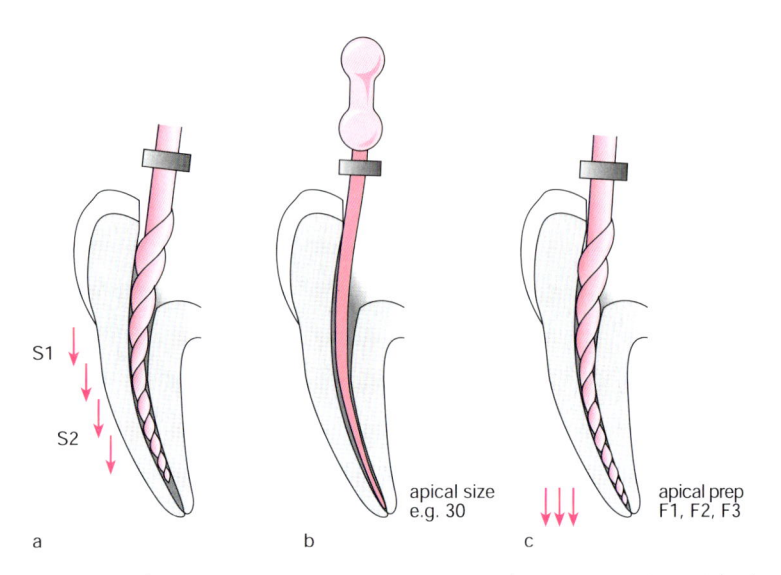

Creating the Conditions for Periapical Health

Fig 6-21 Typical ProTaper preparation. **(a)** Crown-down preparation with Shaper 1, then Shaper 2 at 300rpm. This continues until the apical 1-2mm is reached. **(b)** Apical gauging with standard NiTi instruments. **(c)** Completion of apical preparation with Finisher 1, 2, and 3 according to canal diameter.

Non-tapered NiTi Rotary Systems

A fundamentally different approach is presented by Lightspeed, with features including 22 instruments from size 20-100, with half sizes, all incorporating:
- non-cutting pilot tips (Fig 6-22)
- short cutting heads of 0.5-2mm
- narrow, flexible, non-cutting shanks
- rotation at 750-2000rpm.

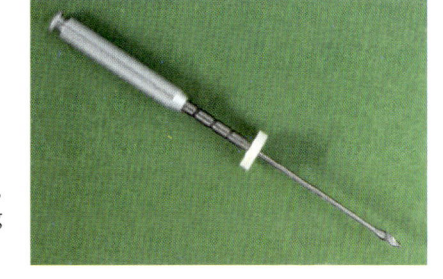

Fig 6-22 Lightspeed, featuring a narrow, taperless, flexible shank, short cutting head and non-cutting pilot tip.

Creating the Conditions for Periapical Health

Preparation begins apically because taperless Lightspeed is uniquely able to gauge canal diameter before flaring.

Typical preparation (Fig 6-23)
- Negotiate canals with a standard size 15 file and determine working length (Fig 6-23a). Canal entrances can be flared with Gates if desired.

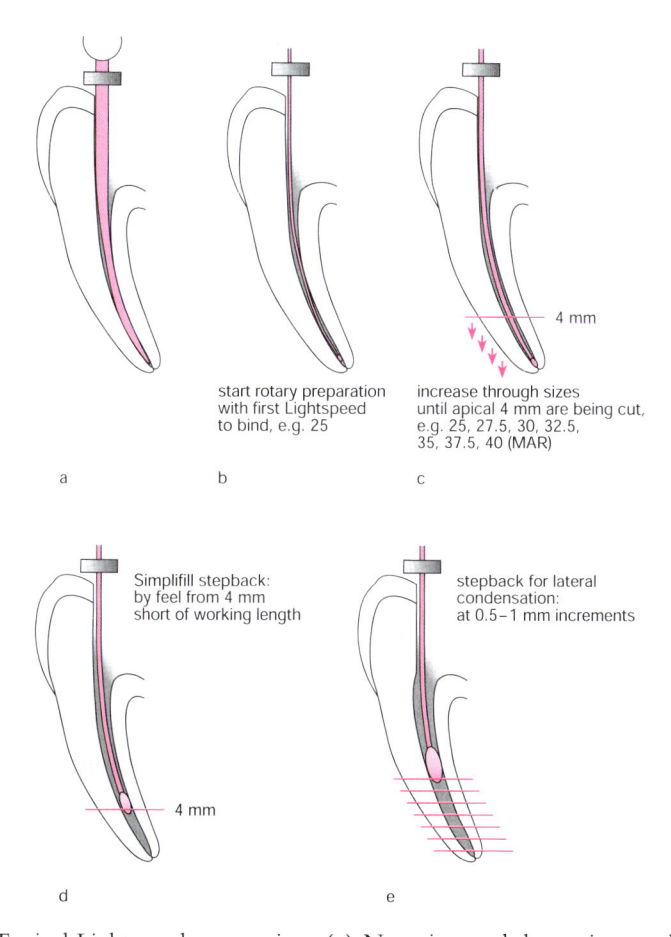

Fig 6-23 Typical Lightspeed preparation. **(a)** Negotiate and determine working length with a standard size 15 file. **(b)** Hand-fit Lightspeed until an instrument binds short of working length. Commence rotary preparation with this instrument and increase through half-sizes. **(c)** Continue until the apical 4mm is being cut. This is the Master Apical Rotary. **(d)** Step back commences 4mm from working length for Lightspeed Simplifill obturation. **(e)** Traditional step back for cold lateral condensation.

- Hand-fit Lightspeed instruments until one binds short of working length (Fig 6-23b).
- Commence rotary preparation with the first binding instrument, sweeping gently into the canal and pecking to nibble dentine as resistance is met. Immediately the instrument reaches working length, sweep it from the canal.
- Continue through half sizes, advancing instruments with pecking motion to working length.
- When an instrument is reached which requires pecking motions during the apical 4mm of the canal, apical preparation is complete (Fig 6-23c). This is the Master Apical Rotary (MAR), and is usually larger than for other techniques.
- The amount of flare depends on obturation technique.
- For Lightspeed Simplifill sectional GP obturation (see Fig 7-8), a parallel 4mm apical preparation and little further enlargement are required. Step back commences 4mm from working length and is completed with just 2 or 3 more instruments which feel to be cutting (Fig 6-23d).
- For cold lateral or warm vertical condensation, more flare is needed and step back is at 0.5-1mm intervals from the apex using instruments which feel to be cutting at the desired level (Fig 6-23e).
- Irrigation is recommended every third instrument and recapitulation to the working length occurs only at the end of preparation with the MAR.

Lightspeed is the most flexible NiTi system and its fragile appearance belies its durability. Large apical preparations are claimed to clean the apical third better than other methods, and conservative tapers may preserve more dentine.

The Pros and Cons of Rotary NiTi

Pros
Rotary NiTi has been a revolution. Amongst its many advantages are:
- Consistent, high-quality canal tapers (Fig 6-24).
- Unsurpassed canal centring, even with greater apical enlargement.
- Simplified, streamlined, rapid preparation protocols.
- Reduced operator fatigue.
- Diminished risk of blockage as material is carried out on the flutes of the rotating instruments.
- Better access for irrigating solutions.

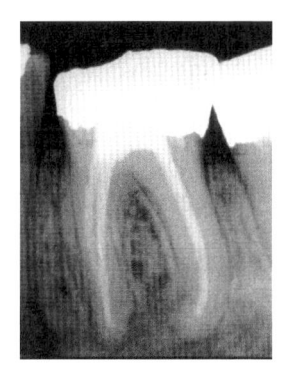

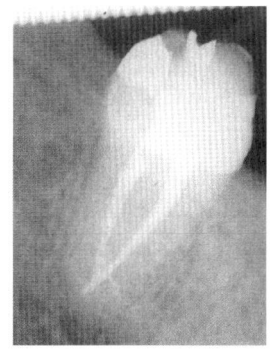

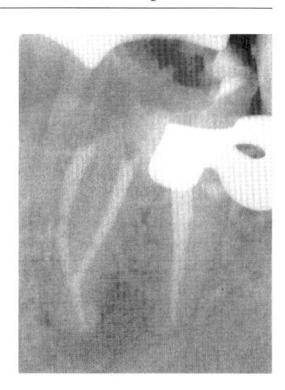

Fig 6-24 Consistent, smooth tapers with a variety of NiTi systems.

Cons

- Costs of start-up hardware and ongoing consumables.
- Reduced preparation times may limit the capacity of sodium hypochlorite to clean canals effectively, though the true impact of this is not known.
- Instrument fracture - a recognised but rare event with proper training, canal exploration, methodical application and disposal of instruments. It may be a small price to pay for an overall increase in quality.
- Rotary instruments, like any other, cannot fully open and clean root canal systems. Just as it is impossible to direct precurved, circumferentially filing instruments into all regions of an oval, curved canal, so NiTi rotaries cannot be steered. The best they can do is concentrically enlarge certain regions, leaving uninstrumented recesses (see Fig 6-2) which will always require thorough irrigation, ideally with sodium hypochlorite and the help of ultrasound.

Which System Is Best?

Marketing information is rife, but there is little evidence to suggest that any NiTi system out-performs others in important areas such as safety and clinical outcome. New NiTi rotary users should therefore sample a variety of techniques in the laboratory to discover which work best in their hands, and all should review their cases and keep a watchful eye on the emerging literature.

The Single-/Multiple-visit Dilemma

Controversy surrounds the merits of single- or multiple-visit treatment. Rotary NiTi heightens the debate as single-visit treatment is now technically possible for most dentists, even in molars.

Canal status may be critical:
- Teeth without apical periodontitis contain few microorganisms, and there is consensus that single-visit treatment is best to preserve an infection-free environment and periapical health.
- Teeth with apical periodontitis contain large numbers of microorganisms, and the question remains whether a single episode of cleaning and shaping kills enough of them or whether an inter-appointment dressing and second-visit irrigation give a more predictable outcome.

A definitive answer cannot be given and the approach adopted must be a matter of outlook, philosophy and practice set-up. Microorganisms cause apical periodontitis, and we should do all we can to kill as many as possible. Intracanal medicaments can help in that process. Patients should always be discharged with advice to expect minor discomfort which may require simple analgesia for up to 48 hours.

Conclusions

- Contemporary manual and mechanical methods are rational because they eliminate most procedural errors and allow predictable, high-quality, concentric enlargement of major canals to the apical constriction.
- Uninstrumented recesses and secondary canal ramifications will always demand the use of antimicrobial irrigants and medicaments.
- There is little evidence to single out any particular technique as best, and debate continues on the desirability of single- or multiple-visit care.

Further Reading

Ruddle CJ. Cleaning and shaping the root canal system. In: Cohen S, Burns RC (Eds.) Pathways of the Pulp. 8th ed. St Louis: Mosby, 2002:231-291.

Spangberg LSW. Endodontic treatment of teeth without apical periodontitis. In: Orstavik D, Pitt Ford TR (Eds.) Essential Endodontology. Prevention and Treatment of Apical Periodontitis. Oxford: Blackwell Science, 1998:211-241.

Sundqvist G, Figdor D. Endodontic treatment of teeth with apical periodontitis. In: Orstavik D, Pitt Ford TR (Eds.) Essential Endodontology. Prevention and Treatment of Apical Periodontitis. Oxford: Blackwell Science, 1998:242-277.

Chapter 7
Preserving the Healing Environment

Aim

To describe methods of preserving a healthy intracanal environment by obliteration with root canal filling material and coronal protection from the oral flora.

Outcome

After studying this chapter, readers should understand the role of the root filling and coronal seal in preserving a clean, health-compatible pulp space. They should also understand the practicalities of obturation with a variety of materials including cold and thermally softened gutta percha and sealer.

Why Fill Root Canals?

Canal preparation eliminates microorganisms and substrate and provides the necessary conditions for periapical health. Many have witnessed substantial healing following preparation alone and questioned whether root fillings are needed (Fig 1-8). Strictly, they are not, provided the internal environment of the tooth remains clean and microbe free. Faced with a similar challenge, a periodontist may recommend regular internal plaque control, irrigation and perhaps the installation of a sustained-release antimicrobial device. Regrettably, repeated entry for environment-preserving "maintenance therapy" is not possible in endodontics since root canal treated teeth must be restored. It is therefore difficult to imagine, in practical terms, how a clean canal system can be preserved without filling it.

The principal role of the filling is to provide a fluid and microbe-tight seal of all coronal, apical and lateral portals of exchange:
- preventing new infection from the oral cavity and
- imprisoning, denying nutrients and space to multiply for any organisms left after preparation.

The coronal restoration is as important as the root filling in achieving these goals; neither will deliver alone.

When Should Root Canals Be Filled?

- When they have been cleaned as thoroughly as possible.
- When they have been shaped for optimal seal.
- When there is enough time to achieve a quality seal (depending on the method, this may not be very long).

For those practising multiple-visit treatment, reassuring signs of adequate preparation include:
- the absence of pain
- the disappearance of sinus tracts.

In single- and multiple-visit treatment, it must be possible to dry the canal.

Incorporating blood or serum:
- compromises seal
- provides rich nutrients and growing-space for microorganisms.

How Should a Root Canal System Be Filled?

The ideal system would introduce a:
- perfectly biocompatible
- perfectly sealing
- permanently antimicrobial
- non-deteriorating

material into every ramification of the root canal system without it ever escaping into surrounding tissues. Partial and total removal would be similarly simple and complete.

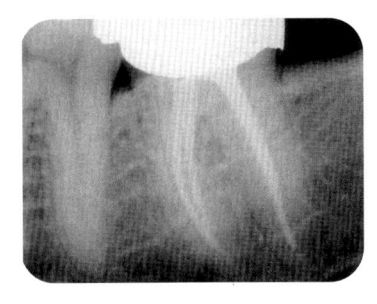

Fig 7-1 Not ideal, but a root filling likely to keep the canal system clean and win clinical success.

It is reassuring that whilst current methods fall short of this ideal; such stringent performance is not needed for predictable clinical success. In fact, excellent outcomes can be expected if all major root canals are prepared and densely filled with bland materials to within 2mm of root-end (Fig 7-1).

Currently, this almost universally involves cold or warm compaction of a rubber material (gutta percha) with a fluid sealer cement.

The Role of Filling Components

Gutta percha provides the bulk of a root filling. It is:
- inexpensive, versatile and easy to handle
- stable and non-deteriorating
- adequately biocompatible
- non-supportive of microbial growth
- capable of adaptation with pressure, solvents and heat
- simple to remove for post-space and re-treatment.

However, it does not seal well on its own and must always be used with a sealer.

Sealer cement acts as a gasket and provides the seal. During compaction, it flows to fill irregularities and provides a tight interface with canal walls. Sealers may also:
- lubricate the glide-path of gutta percha into the canal
- actively suppress microbial growth
- promote hard-tissue repair at the root end.

Slow-setting materials are preferred which allow:
- time for adequate gutta percha compaction, even in the presence of humidity and heat
- continued flow during setting to counter shrinkage forces which might otherwise pull the material away from canal walls and break the seal.

Surprisingly little is known about the relative clinical performance of root canal sealers (Table 7-1), and no material has been convincingly shown to provide superior short- or long-term clinical outcomes. Selection is usually based on nothing more than ease of handling and personal preference.

The properties of gutta percha and sealer are generally held to be optimised by maximising the volume of rubber and minimising the volume of sealer (Fig 7-2). This can be achieved by cold compaction or after softening with heat.

Table 7-1 **Examples of commercially available slow-setting root canal sealers and some of their properties.**

Category	Comments	Examples
Zinc oxide/eugenol-based	The most widely used globally. Irritant to tissues in the unset state but resorbable and inert when set. Contains antimicrobial eugenol.	TubliSeal® extended working time (Kerr) Pulp Canal Sealer® extended working time (Kerr)
Calcium hydroxide-based	Biocompatible and may be osteoregenerative, but concerns over long-term solubility.	Apexit® (Ivoclar) Sealapex® (Kerr)
Resin-based	Popular in Europe, with long working times and easy to remove with solvents. Irritant until set and may resorb slowly if extruded.	AH Plus® (Dentsply)
Glass-ionomer-based	Early promise of enhanced seal and root reinforcement has not been realised. Pre-encapsulation leads to waste. Can be very difficult to remove for post-space and retreatment.	Ketac Endo® (ESPE)
Silicone-based	Promising early research supports their use.	ReokoSeal® (Reoko)

Fig 7-2 Optimising material properties by increasing the volume of rubber and reducing the volume of sealer: **(a)** Single cones in a large volume of sealer. **(b)** Multiple-point cold lateral condensation. **(c)** Thermoplastic obturation.

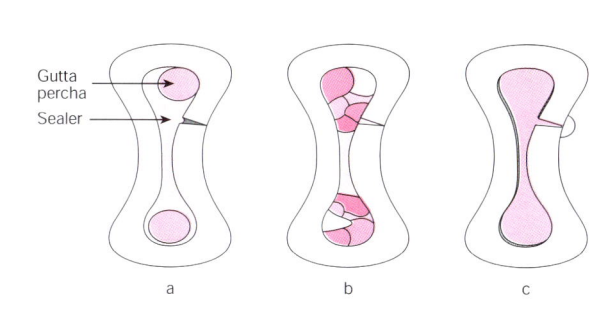

Cold Compaction of Gutta Percha with Sealer

1. Cold lateral condensation
Principles: Multiple cones of gutta percha compacted to form a dense core with thin interposing and surrounding films of sealer (Fig 7-2b). Condensation is performed with a smooth, tapered "spreader" which acts like a wedge to squeeze the rubber laterally under vertical pressure (Fig 7-3), not by pushing it sideways like a root-splitting crow bar.

Preparing to fill
All condensing tools (spreaders and pluggers) should be tried in the prepared canal to make sure they will be able to work at the required level. A correct spreader should pass to the root terminus if it is to compact the filling into the apical seat and throughout its length.

ISO or non-ISO spreaders?
This is a matter of personal preference. Highly tapered, non-ISO spreaders (e.g. medium-fine, fine-medium) generate greater lateral force than .02 tapered ISO instruments, but more dentine should not be removed to accommodate them.

Stainless steel or NiTi?
NiTi spreaders are especially useful in curved canals, penetrating deeper and placing less stress on canal walls.

Accessory cone selection
When a spreader is removed from the canal, it leaves a space of its own size and taper. Accessory cones should match or be slightly narrower than the spreader so they will bottom-out in the spreader track and avoid air voids.

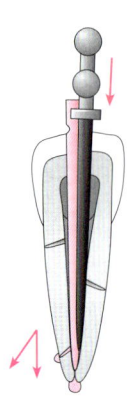

Fig 7-3 Cold lateral condensation generates lateral force by axial loading of a wedge-like spreader. The greater its taper, the greater the lateral component of force. There is always a vertical component of condensation which is increased if the spreader has a flat, rather than pointed tip.

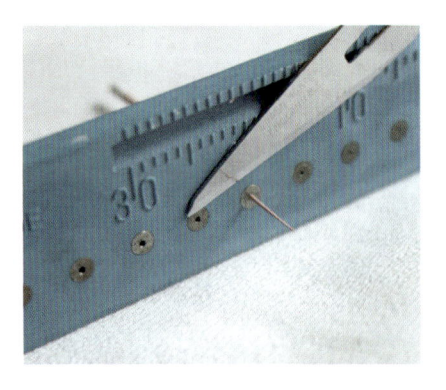

Fig 7-4 Customising gutta percha cone tip diameter with a gauge (Maillefer/Dentsply) and scalpel.

Master cone fit

ISO or non-ISO cones can be fitted to the apical preparation. ISO cones usually size match the master apical file, but it should be noted that standardisation is not always as accurate as we would wish. Position of fit is more important than nominal size match. Non-ISO medium-fine or fine-medium cones are suitable for most conventionally prepared canals. They may traverse curved canals better than ISO cones which can sometimes buckle, and have less tendency to slide through the apex if apical resistance form is not ideal.

Tip diameter can be customised with a commercially available gauge and sharp scalpel (Fig 7-4). Master cones are tried in irrigant-moistened canals to lubricate their path in the same way as the sealer will. If a well-fitting spreader is available, the master cone should fit to within 0.5mm of the apical terminus.

Short master cones may be due to
- apical obstruction
- tip-size incompatibility.

Apical obstruction with cutting debris is removed by irrigating and repeating the apical preparation with Balanced-Force motion, finishing with a quarter-clockwise turn before withdrawal to load the apical flutes of the file with debris "apical clearing". Apical obstructions due to ledging usually require gentle canal filing to remove wall defects, or employing an over-curved GT hand file to bypass and plane away irregularities.

Tip size incompatibility is often overcome by trying another cone from the same pack, or re-trimming another non-ISO cone to a smaller tip size. Long master cones usually occur because of inadequate apical resistance form. This is usually a function of inaccurate working length determination, or of employing a clockwise-rotating file motion at root-end. The stop should be redefined at a shorter length, or a non-ISO cone trimmed and fitted which will have less risk of compaction beyond root-end.

Drying the canal
Final drying is done by aspiration with the irrigation needle and syringe, and wicking remaining moisture with paper points. Some finish the drying process with a final flush of absolute alcohol.

Sealer
Sealer can now be mixed in accordance with the manufacturer's instructions and accessory cones arranged ready for use.

The filling process (Fig 7-5)
Sealer application
Sealer should coat all walls of the canal. This is most consistently achieved by:
- filling the canal with a lentulospiral paste filler
- insertion on a file before ultrasonic activation.

Incremental addition with a small hand file, inserted and turned anticlockwise during advance into the canal, is the commonest but least effective method.

Most of the excess sealer will displace coronally during condensation, though small amounts may find themselves extruded through apical or lateral portals of exit.

Master cone insertion (Fig 7-5a)
A lightly coated master cone is now slowly advanced with slight up-down pumping motion and firmly seated in the apical part of the canal. If canals are confluent, master cones should be inserted into both consecutively.

Spreader insertion (Fig 7-5b)
The measured spreader is then inserted deep with 1-3 Kg vertical finger pressure. Gutta percha requires several seconds to deform at canal temperature, and the spreader is held in place for at least ten seconds before watch-winding rotation to free it before removal. Energising the spreader with ultrasound or a reciprocating handpiece can warm and assist flow of the gutta percha.

Accessory cone insertion and build-up of the filling (Fig 7-5c)
Immediately on removing the spreader, an accessory cone, lightly coated in sealer, is slid to the base of the spreader track.

The spreader is inserted deep once again, and the process continued. Compression is taking place predominantly at the tip of the spreader as it walks progressively out of the tapered canal. Condensation and insertion of gutta percha continues until the spreader will reach no deeper than 2-3mm into the canal (i.e. beyond the cementum/enamel junction). There is no benefit in continuing to the cavosurface of the access cavity.

Severing with heat (Fig 7-5d)
Cold lateral condensation is never just that. Material is always severed deep with heat from a:
- red-hot heat carrier
- battery-operated "touch 'n' heat" instrument.

After cutting off, the warmed mass of gutta percha is firmly condensed with a plugger to improve adaptation and consolidate the fill. Softening extends up to 5mm into a mass of warmed gutta percha, and vertical condensation of this sort can exert an influence deep into the canal system.

Foundations
Cold lateral condensation can stand alone, or form the foundation for:
- continued warm vertical condensation, with deeper waves of heating and packing to improve density and adaptation
- thermomechanical compaction, where a rotary condenser creates frictional heat and carries in softened material (Fig 7-6).

Preserving the Healing Environment

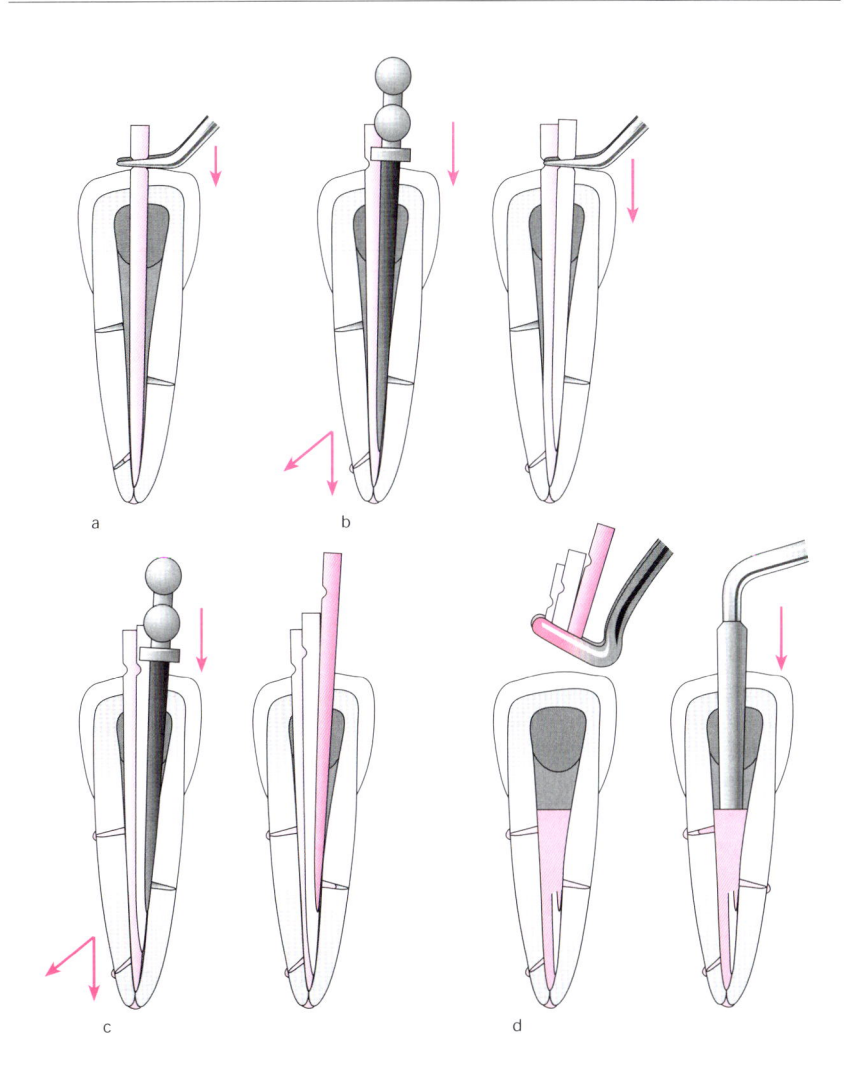

Fig 7-5 Cold lateral condensation. **(a)** Sliding the master cone home lightly coated with sealer. **(b)** Spreader application, loaded vertically with 1-3Kg force. The spreader remains in place for ten seconds before watch-winding, withdrawal and insertion of an accessory cone. **(c)** Progressive application and build-up as the spreader walks out of the canal. Accessory cones should slide to length and bottom-out in the spreader track. Packing continues until the spreader can reach no more than 2-3mm into the canal. **(d)** Severing deep with heat. Heat transmits up to 5mm through the mass of gutta percha and can be condensed to improve the filling and make space for the restoration.

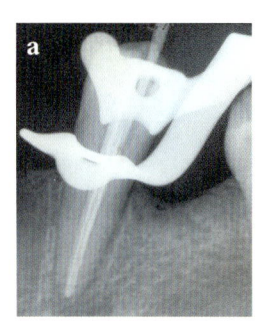

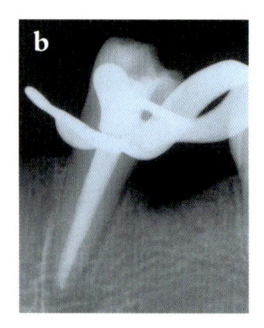

Fig 7-6 Thermomechanical compaction. **(a)** A wide canal partially filled by cold lateral condensation. **(b)** The same canal after five seconds of thermomechanical compaction. Excess material outside the canal was warmed and fed-in by the mechanical compactor.

At least 3mm of space should be available for a sealing provisional or permanent restoration.

The gold standard
Cold lateral condensation remains the gold standard obturation technique against which all others should be evaluated. Those who practise cold lateral condensation well have nothing to be ashamed of. If they wish to supplement their technique, that is well and good, but there is no method shown to provide better long-term clinical outcomes at this time.

2. Lightspeed Simplifill (Fig 7-7)
Single-cone obturation techniques fell out of favour when it was realised that curved canals could not be prepared to a circular cross-section with conventional instruments. Equally, large volumes of sealer have been shunned because of:
- difficult length control
- erratic density
- setting contraction in large volumes of material which may disrupt close wall adaptation and seal.

Simplifill challenges convention by fitting a parallel section of gutta percha into a circular apical 4mm Lightspeed preparation before backfilling with sealer.

Try-in
A size-matched Simplifill apical plug is tried in the moist canal (Fig 7-8a).

Preserving the Healing Environment

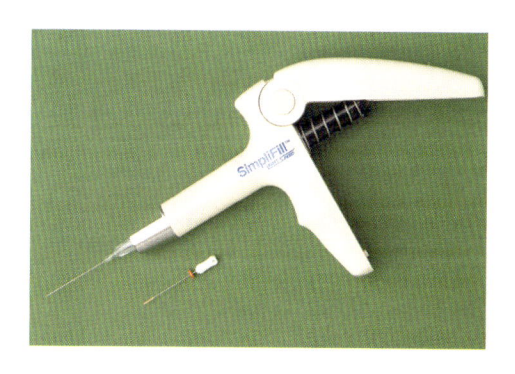

Fig 7-7 Lightspeed Simplifill apical tip and backfill syringe.

Slight resistance should be felt as it advances into the apical preparation and it should not be finally driven home if apical resistance is felt. The device is removed without twisting and dried.

Seating the apical plug
After drying and sealer application (AHPlus or Ketac Endo are recommended), the tip is slid with some pressure to full working length (Fig 7-8b). The metal carrier is unscrewed anticlockwise, leaving the apical preparation "corked" with a gutta percha plug (Fig 7-8c).

Backfill
Sealer delivered with a 27 gauge needle and applicator gun to backfill from the apical plug, and a single gutta percha cone inserted to provide a ready pathway for retreatment or post space preparation (Fig 7-8d). Alternatively, the space can be compacted more densely with laterally condensed gutta percha.

It remains to be seen if this simple system which exploits the concentricity of NiTi preparation performs as well as other techniques clinically (Fig 7-8e). There is no reason why it should not.

Warm Gutta Percha Techniques

Anatomical complexity means that few canal systems are completely free of bacteria at the time of obturation. It is therefore rational to work harder to imprison bacteria remaining in canal ramifications by thermally softening gutta percha to improve its flow. As a result, more secondary anatomy can be demonstrated (Fig 7-9), which may be important to dentists because:
- they may feel they are filling canal systems more completely

Preserving the Healing Environment

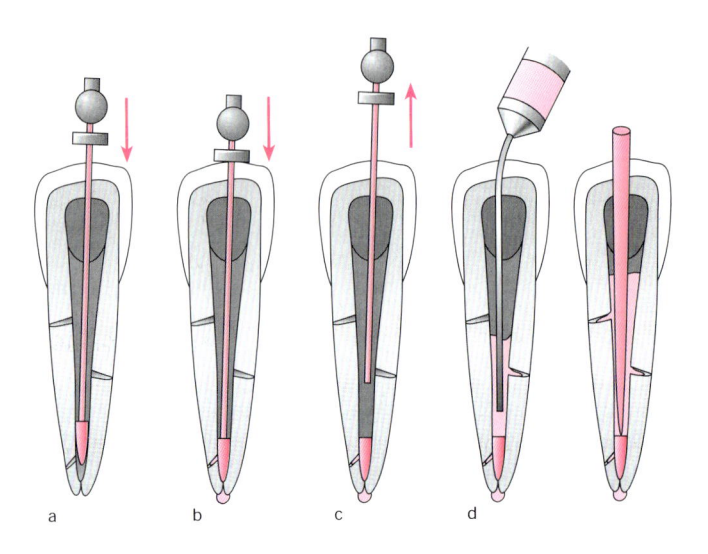

Fig 7-8 Lightspeed Simplifill technique. **(a)** Trying an apical tip in an irrigant-moistened canal. It should meet resistance but should not be fully seated. **(b)** Seating the apical tip fully in a sealer-coated canal. **(c)** Removal of the carrier, leaving a tightly fitting apical plug of gutta percha. **(d)** Backfill with sealer. Gutta percha can be added if desired to provide a path for retreatment or post-preparation.

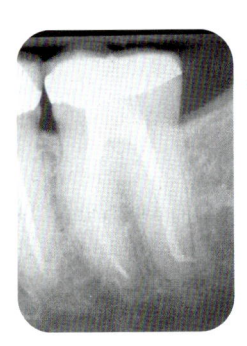

(e) Technically satisfactory outcome. In common with many techniques, long-term outcomes are not known.

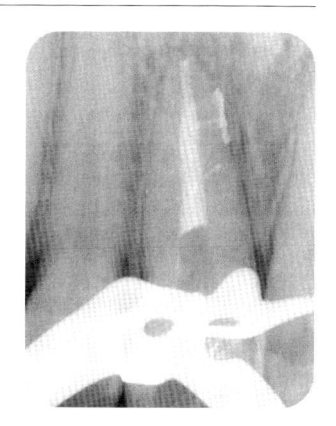

Fig 7-9 A pleasing display of secondary anatomy, but does it matter? (Courtesy G V Seccombe).

- the postoperative radiograph may reveal exciting surprises to enliven their practice - "the thrill of the fill"
- the achievement of a complex postoperative "look" may imply greater mastery of technique than cases in which just the main canals are densely filled.

There is currently little evidence that demonstrating secondary anatomy has any real impact on healing outcome, but all the points listed are laudable enough in maintaining interest and working to do our best for patients.

1. Warm vertical condensation – multiple wave
The traditional Schilder technique involves repeated episodes of heating and compaction.
- The preparation usually has a wide taper, with an apical control zone, rather than a stop.
- At least three pluggers of decreasing tip diameter are needed (Fig 7-10). They should be tried in the canal to confirm depth of penetration. The smallest should extend no closer than 5mm from working length (Fig 7-11a).
- Cone fit is usually with a cone of similar taper to the preparation (e. g., .06 taper), trimmed to give slight tug-back 0.5mm short of working length. Fine-tuning of filling length is sometimes achieved by noting a constant drying point in a preparation without a stop. In canals which are confluent, the straightest path should be used to cone-fit the apex. The other canal can then be cone-fit to the point of confluence (Fig 7-11b).
- After drying and lightly coating the canal with sealer, the master cone is seated to length (Fig 7-11b). In confluent canals, the other cone is seated

Preserving the Healing Environment

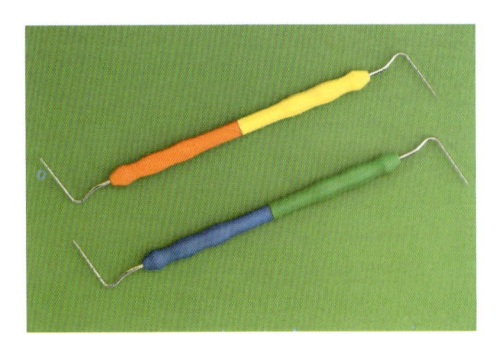

Fig 7-10 Pluggers for warm vertical condensation (Maillefer/Dentsply).

at the same time. Hydraulic pressure during vertical compaction can dramatically "shoot" sealer through the apex. Excess should be avoided.
- Heat can be supplied by a heat-carrier, warmed red–hot over a bunsen burner, or with a touch 'n' heat. Gutta percha is severed below canal entrance level and pressure applied with the first cold plugger (Fig 7-11c). Care should be taken not to drive the plugger too deep and make direct wall contact which can generate damaging wedge-like forces.
- Second and successive waves of heating remove bites of softened gutta percha from the canal (there is no need to be alarmed), whilst pluggers advance deeper into the apically narrowing preparation (Fig 7-11d,e). The process of heating/removal and compaction continues until the apical 5–7mm are reached.
- Downpack is now complete and the apex "corked" with well-adapted material (Fig 7-11e). The tapering apical preparation should have prevented movement of gutta percha beyond the apex provided that heat was kept out of the apical 5mm. It is expected that material will have been forced into all secondary anatomy during the downpack, and unless a post is planned, the empty space should now be back-filled.
- Back-fill is achieved most quickly with an injection-moulded gutta percha gun system. After adding more sealer, the needle is advanced and held for a few seconds to warm the canal and surface of the apical plug before passively injecting, welding the new gutta percha to the apical increment and rapidly filling the dead space (Fig 7-11f). Cold pluggers are again used to counteract shrinkage in each 3-4mm length of material deposited. Alternatively, 3-4mm lengths of tapered gutta percha can be added to the canal with a little sealer, heated as previously and packed apically, progressively walking out of the canal.

This sectional technique is more time-consuming, technique-sensitive and prone to voids than the more expensive gun method.

Preserving the Healing Environment

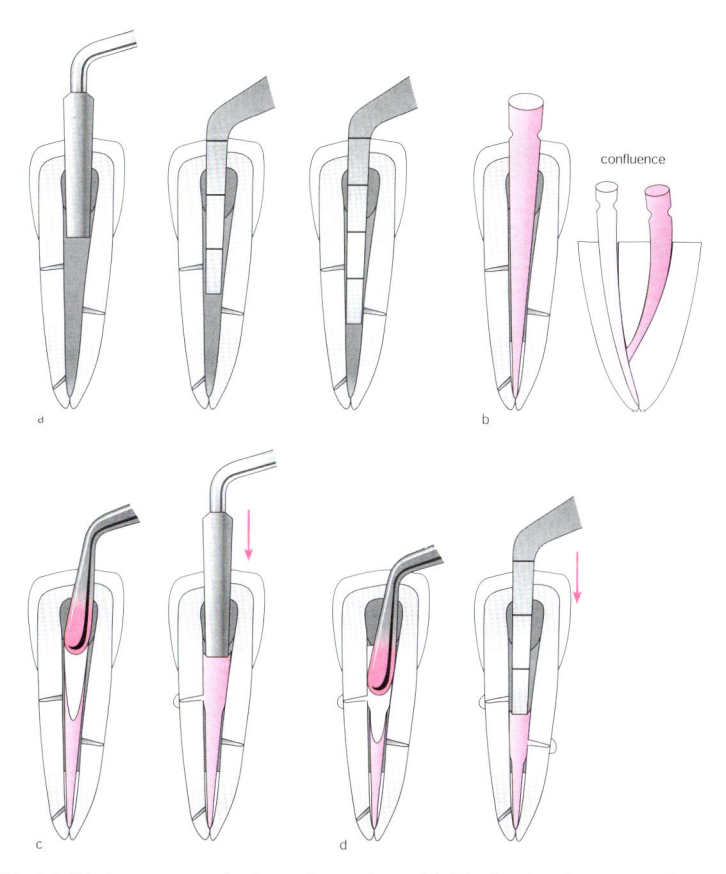

Fig 7-11 Multiple wave vertical condensation. **(a)** Trying in pluggers. The smallest should reach 5mm from working length. **(b)** Seating the master cones. With confluent canals, the straightest path is used for the apical cone, and the second cone trimmed and inserted to the confluence. **(c)** First wave of heating and compaction. **(d)** Second wave of heating and compaction.

2. Warm vertical condensation – single wave

Warm vertical condensation has been transformed by the Buchanan System (System B®) heat source with its series of tips (Fig 7-12) which:
- heat instantly from the tip when activated
- cool almost as rapidly on de-activation.

This means that the same tip can be used as both heat source and cold plugger, largely eliminating the need for multiple applications of heat and compaction.

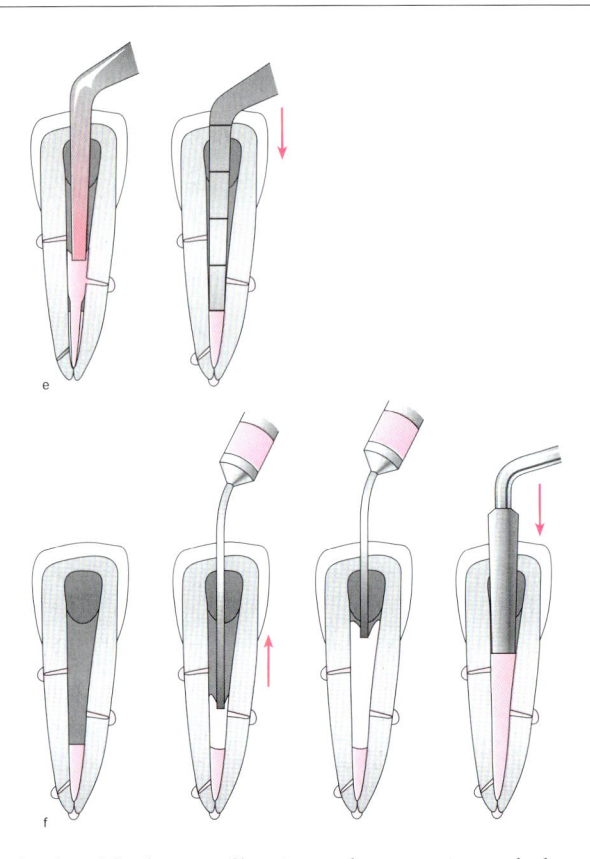

Fig 7-11(e) Third and final wave of heating and compaction seals the apex. **(f)** Post space is now available, or the canal can be back-filled with a gun system.

- Canal preparation and cone fit is exactly as described for the multiple wave technique.
- One heater/plugger tip is selected for each canal which will extend deep and bind against the walls approximately 5–7mm from working length (Fig 7-13a). They are made from soft metal and will bend into curves. It is also wise to pre-fit a regular stainless steel or Buchanan NiTi plugger should this become necessary.
- Sealer is lightly coated on the walls and master cone, which is seated to length.
- Downpack is in one fluid movement with the System B® heat source set to 200°C. The warm tip takes two seconds to advance through softened material to approximately 2mm short of the binding point (Fig 7-13b). The heat

Preserving the Healing Environment

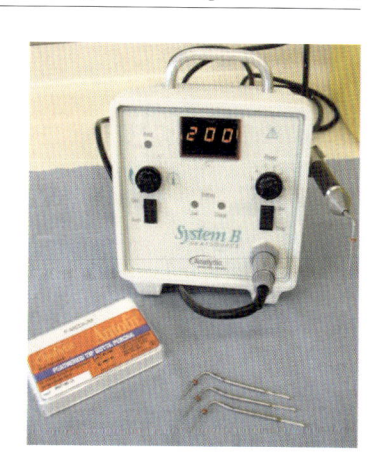

Fig 7-12 The versatile System B® heat source with its variety of heater/plugger tips.

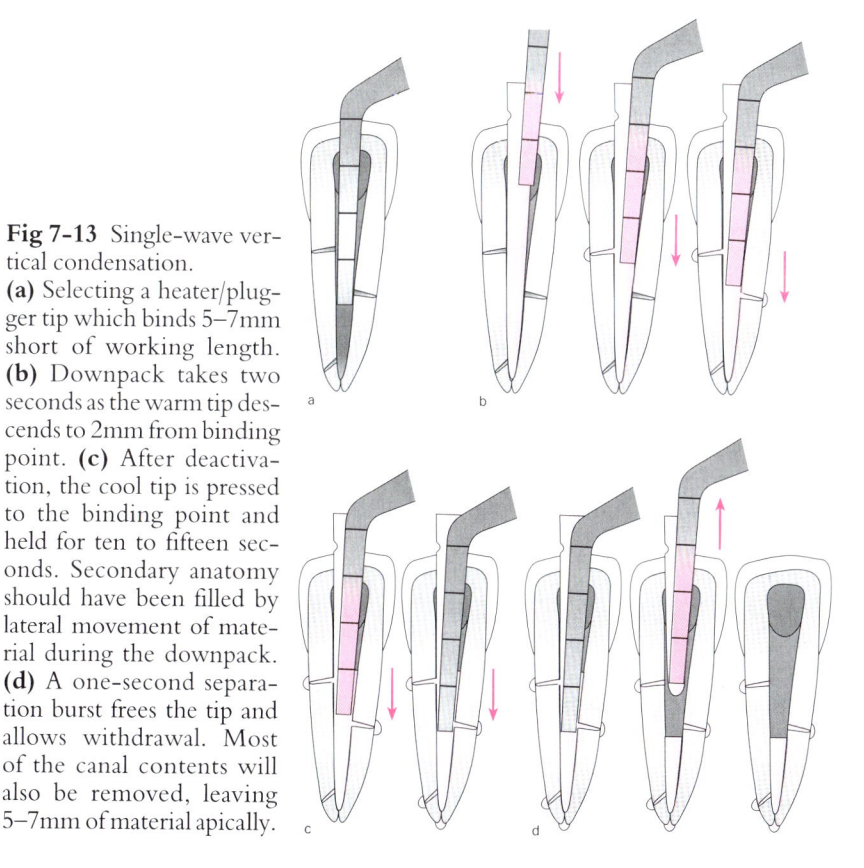

Fig 7-13 Single-wave vertical condensation.
(a) Selecting a heater/plugger tip which binds 5–7mm short of working length.
(b) Downpack takes two seconds as the warm tip descends to 2mm from binding point. **(c)** After deactivation, the cool tip is pressed to the binding point and held for ten to fifteen seconds. Secondary anatomy should have been filled by lateral movement of material during the downpack.
(d) A one-second separation burst frees the tip and allows withdrawal. Most of the canal contents will also be removed, leaving 5–7mm of material apically.

103

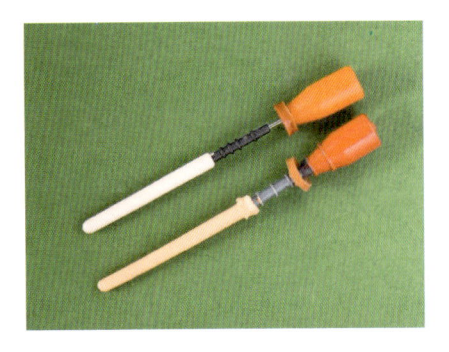

Fig 7-14 Gutta percha/carrier systems.

is de-activated and pressure continued to advance the cooling tip to binding point (Fig 7-13c). Pressure is maintained for ten to fifteen seconds as the apical plug of gutta percha cools and shrinks.
- Separation burst and withdrawal completes the downpack. Filling materials will have cooled in contact with the heater/plugger tip which can only be removed by activating the heat again for a one-second "separation burst" (Fig 7-13d). Gutta percha lying coronal to the binding point is removed, attached to the tip.
- Consolidation of the apical plug is achieved with the stainless steel or NiTi Buchanan plugger.
- Back-fill is then completed as before. If the System B® heat source is used for heating increments of back-fill gutta percha, its temperature can usefully be reduced to approximately 100°C.

The System B heat source is the most versatile and user-friendly device for warm compaction, either in a pure single wave technique, or to revise and consolidate any other gutta percha filling. Battery-operated heaters of this sort are predictable and do away with the dangers and inconsistencies of carrying red-hot instruments to the mouth.

3. Carrier systems
Carrier systems such as Thermafil® (Maillefer/Dentsply) and Softcore® (Septodont) (Fig 7-14) promise speed and simplicity in thermoplastic obturation.
- Preparation should be a smooth .06 taper and verified by trying in a blank plastic carrier/condenser, which should freely reach the canal terminus (Fig 7-15a).
- Heating must be complete and uniform for predictable flow, and the correct oven and heating time are essential.

Preserving the Healing Environment

- Carrier insertion should occur smoothly and rapidly in a well-prepared, lightly sealer-coated canal (Fig 7-15b). Excess sealer may shoot apically like the contents of a syringe and should be avoided.
- Cooling shrinkage should be countered by walking around the carrier with a cold plugger.
- After one to two minutes of cooling and compaction, the handle can be removed with a hot instrument or bur (Fig 7-15c). Post preparation is then possible, either with a dedicated high-speed bur or slow-speed Gates Glidden/Peezo drills.

Well done, carriers will deliver pleasing and rapid results, and it is likely that they will perform as well as any other method. However, there are some possible disadvantages:

- Failure to seat. Inadequate initial heating or a moment's distraction during insertion will compromise smooth insertion and flow, with disappointing consequences.
- Stripping of gutta percha from the carrier. If the preparation is not smooth or properly accommodating of the carrier, gutta percha may be wiped away during insertion, leaving a bare plastic core with severely compromised sealing ability at the apex.
- Inability to revise. In the event of disappointment, the presence of the plastic carrier thwarts any attempt to revise or advance the fill. This is in contrast with all-gutta-percha methods which can be revised until satisfied.

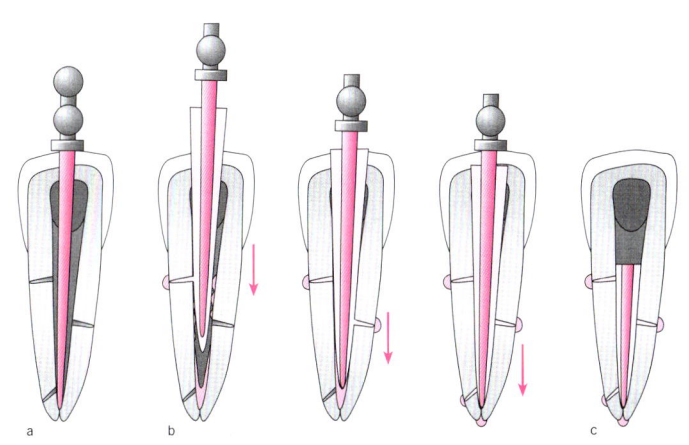

Fig 7-15 Carrier systems. **(a)** Verification of the preparation. **(b)** Seating of the warmed carrier into a lightly sealer-coated canal, smoothly and without delay. **(c)** Severing the handle deep to allow adequate coronal protection.

Preserving the Healing Environment

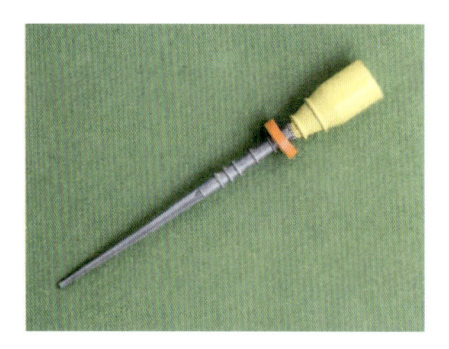

Fig 7-16 V-shaped notch to facilitate removal of Thermafil®.

- Difficult removal. Retrieval of a part-seated carrier can be a time-consuming challenge. Thermafil® devices incorporate a groove for entry of instruments (Fig 7-16), but retrieval is still generally difficult.
- Postoperative pain. Carrier systems appear to be associated with increased postoperative pain, which usually resolves within 24 to 48 hours. Explanations may include extrusion of canal contents due to the great hydraulic pressures generated.
- Confluent canals present a special challenge. Excess gutta percha and sealer extrude into the second canal and may prevent full seating of the next carrier.

Positive indications include the very long or severely curved canal where the carriage of heat and compaction by any other method may be difficult (Fig 7-17).

The Challenge of the Open Apex

Open root-ends commonly result from:
- apical inflammatory root resorption in teeth with long-standing apical periodontitis
- over-instrumentation beyond the root terminus
- failure of root formation after childhood trauma (Fig 7-18a).

Regardless of the aetiology, open root ends present a challenge for controlled and well-sealing obturation. Traditional approaches have included:
- repeated calcium hydroxide dressings to grow a calcific apical barrier
- generation of an apical barrier with calcium hydroxide powder to pack gutta percha against
- customising large gutta percha cones with heat or solvents
- root-end surgery.

Preserving the Healing Environment

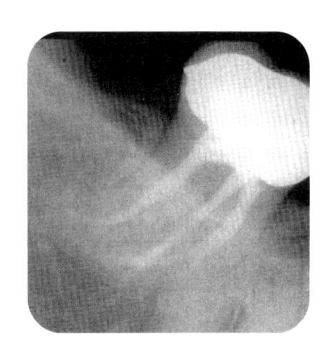

Fig 7-17 A positive indication for carrier obturation, where heat and condensing instruments may be unable to penetrate deeply enough.

Increasingly, this and other types of repair (including perforation repairs) are achieved non-surgically with Mineral Trioxide Aggregate (MTA), an exciting material:
- based on Portland building cement
- mixed to a stiff, gritty consistency with water
- packed and vibrated in increments with long pluggers and paper points to deliver unsurpassed sealing and bioregenerative results in the apical periodontium (Fig 7-18b).

The filling should be kept moist by gentle overlaying with moistened cotton wool and a tight coronal seal, and will set within a few hours. Setting should be confirmed by inspecting and probing the material at least 24 hours after placement and before definitive resoration of the tooth.
MTA is emerging as an exceptional material in non-surgical and surgical endodontics, and is likely to develop many new roles and formulations. However, applications are currently limited by poor handling characteristics (crumbly, and with behaviour like pumice and water), and the propensity to tattoo tissues in aesthetically sensitive areas. Until these properties are improved, it is unlikely to displace gutta percha and sealer as the material of choice for most filling applications.

Postoperative Warnings

Although the likelihood of serious postoperative flare-up is low, all endodontic patients should be dismissed with the warning that they may experience minor discomfort and require simple analgesia for the next 48 hours. They should also be notified of the importance of getting a root-canal-treated tooth properly restored.

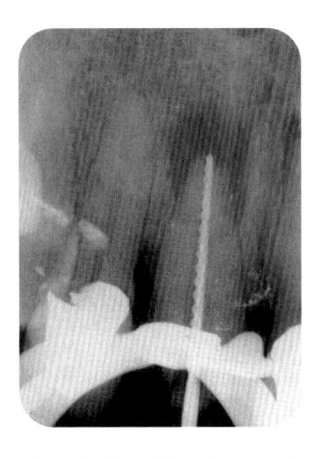

Fig 7-18a The damaged, open apex presents special challenges for controlled obturation.

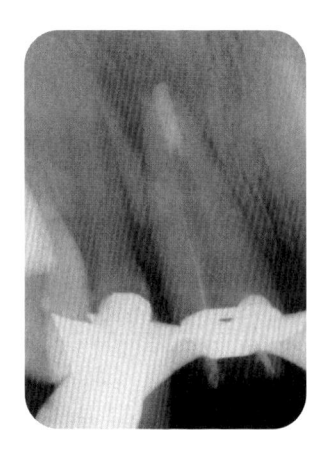

Fig 7-18b completed MTA compaction.

Protection of Root Fillings

For all of our focus on preparation and obturation, it should be remembered that gutta percha/sealer root fillings leak and should be protected from the oral flora. Some studies have shown that the human salivary flora penetrates the full length of a well-compacted root filling within four to 40 days. The spectre of failure should not be underestimated in the excitement of a pleasing root filling. Gutta percha and sealer should be cut back deeply to provide at least 3mm thickness of well-sealing restorative material, adapted with care against the walls of the preparation. Cuspal protection should also be provided for teeth vulnerable to fracture.

Conclusions

- The healthy environment of a prepared root canal will not be sustained longterm without obturation and coronal seal.
- Satisfactory root canal fillings can be achieved in well-prepared canals with gutta percha and sealer compacted by a variety of cold and warm techniques.
- Although there is little evidence currently of improved outcomes, it is rational to assume that techniques better able to obliterate three-dimensionally the pulp canal space are preferable.

- Whilst gutta percha and sealer remains the gold standard, alternatives including MTA are justifiably gaining acceptance in a variety of settings.

Further Reading

Gutmann JL, Witherspoon DE. Obturation of the cleaned and shaped root canal system. In: Cohen S, Burns RC (Eds.) Pathways of the Pulp. 8th ed. St Louis: Mosby, 2002: 293-364.

Root canal obturation. In: Beer R, Baumann MA, Kim S (Eds.) Color Atlas of Dental Medicine. Endodontology. Stuttgart: Thieme, 2000:165-198.

Chapter 8
Success and Failure

Aim
To outline minimalist and more stringent definitions of endodontic success, review factors affecting outcome and develop a rational basis for evaluating treatment at intervals after its completion.

Outcome
After studying this chapter, the reader should have a clearer understanding of factors associated with successful root canal treatment; the signs of progress at intervals after treatment; and the consequences of inadequate infection control.

Defining Outcome
Where you stand on an issue depends on where you sit. Patients, clinicians, academics and healthcare organisations all have an interest in successful therapies, including root canal treatment. Whilst clinical academics usually develop "official" definitions of success and failure, everyone has a working understanding of what they consider acceptable. This can range from a minimalist "uncomplaining patient with tooth still present" to a stringent "histological resolution of inflammation and return of tissues to pristine health". Both extremes may be unreasonable.

Minimalist Definitions of Success
Root canal treatments are often provided for teeth with painful symptoms, but equal numbers are provided for uncomplaining patients, unaware of their necrotic pulp and apical periodontitis. If treatment is offered to prevent and cure disease, it must do more than simply preserve a diseased status quo. Emergence of apical periodontitis, or failure of it to diminish or heal after root canal treatment can only mean that the aetiological agents were inadequately managed and that treatment did not meet its objectives (Fig 8-1).

Stringent Definitions of Success

Histological monitoring of success is equally unrealistic. Even if they were justified, biopsy results would be disappointing, with few treated teeth completely free of periapical inflammatory cells.

Official Definitions

These try to strike a rational middle ground, embracing patient comfort and function as well as reasonable evidence of healing:
- No pain, swelling or other symptoms of endodontic origin.
- No sinus tract of endodontic origin, either through the mucosa or through the periodontal ligament.
- No limitation of chewing function.
- Radiographic evidence of a normal periodontal ligament space around the root.

Guidelines consistently note that a symptom-free periapical lesion which remains unchanged or only diminishes in size cannot be counted as success and most commonly demands further review if not further treatment.

Factors Associated with Success and Failure

Achieving a successful outcome in the terms defined can be influenced by the:
- preoperative condition of the patient and tooth
- treatment provided
- management and maintenance of the tooth after treatment.

Preoperative Condition of the Patient and Tooth

Age, gender and health of the patient
Since apical periodontitis represents a balance between intracanal infection and host defences, it might be assumed that host factors would exert a major influence on treatment outcome. Surprisingly, there is little indication that they do, and there are consequently few contraindications for root canal treatment. However, severely immunocompromised and patients about to undergo radiotherapy to the jaws may not heal as quickly and predictably as others, and extraction with medical liaison is usually the preferred treatment for apical periodontitis in such cases.

Presence of apical periodontitis
This is the single most important factor in studies of endodontic outcome.
- Teeth without apical periodontitis are more likely to maintain apical health after treatment than teeth with apical periodontitis are likely completely to heal.
- Since apical status is important in defining success, teeth without apical periodontitis (irreversible pulpitis cases) are approximately 25% more likely to be successful than cases with pulp necrosis and established apical periodontitis (Fig 8-2 a,b).

There are few studies to show that root canal treatment restores comfort and function more predictably for teeth with or without apical periodontitis.

Size of periapical lesion
Periapical lesions can develop over many years. Lesions >5mm diameter may be expected to fill with bone more slowly than those <5mm diameter. There are, of course, exceptions (Fig 1-8), and large lesions can heal by soft-tissue scarring which may be difficult to distinguish from persistent inflammation.

Condition and position of the tooth
Pulpectomy and root canal treatment predictably relieve symptoms of pulpitis and heal apical periodontitis. There is no convincing evidence that molars and their surrounding tissues are less responsive to treatment than any other tooth. However, factors which may compromise treatment such as:
- coronal breakdown
- anatomical complexity
- difficult access
- calcification
- curvature
- cracks

may be more prevalent or multiply represented in multi-rooted posterior teeth, making their treatment appear less predictable.

Nature of the canal flora or periapical lesion
Most apical lesions are sustained by infections which are disrupted or eliminated by canal preparation. However, there are instances of:
- intracanal infection resistant to normal measures
- extraradicular infections inaccessible to routine procedures
- periapical lesions independent of intracanal infection (see Chapter 1).

These probably represent less than 5% of all cases with apical periodontitis and diagnostics are currently unable to detect them. The smell of a root canal

Success and Failure

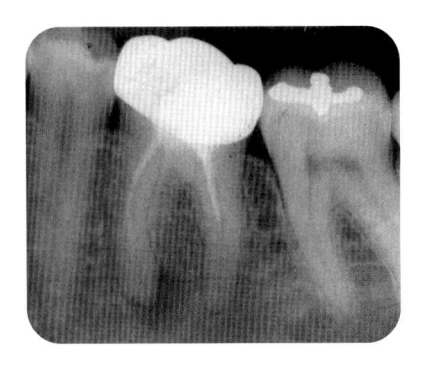

Fig 8-1 A symptom-free case, but can this really represent success?

and the appearance of a lesion's margins (corticated or not) are not prognostic indicators.

The Treatment Provided

Much of this book has been devoted to technical aspects of root canal access, preparation and obturation. It would be reasonable to assume that studies were available to give strong guidance on which techniques promote better healing:
- modest v. increased apical enlargement
- modest v. increased canal taper
- irrigation with weak or strong bleach
- cold lateral condensation v. warm vertical condensation
- demonstration of complex anatomy with filling materials
- choice of root canal sealer
- single- v. multiple-visit treatment.

Regrettably, few procedures have been subjected to randomised clinical trials with follow-up of sufficient duration, and guidelines are only available in the broadest terms.

Quality of the Root Filling

Success is most strongly associated with cases in which the postoperative radiograph shows a root filling:
- contained within the tooth
- extending to within 2mm of the root-end
- with no evidence of empty space apical to, lateral to, or within the body of filling material (Fig 8-3).

It may be realistic to assume that practitioners who strive to achieve these outcomes also embrace other aspects of treatment to control infection.

Persistent Root Canal Infection

The presence of cultivable bacteria in root canals at the time of filling reduces the likelihood of periapical healing from almost 95% to less than 70%. Procedural accidents which deny access to the whole canal for disinfection, such as:
- ledging
- blocking canals with infected debris
- fracturing instruments

are therefore likely to impact heavily on success.

Similarly, accidents which compromise the development of a seal including:
- apical transportation
- destruction of the root terminus by over-instrumentation
- lateral root perforation
- splitting of the root

will foil attempts to preserve a clean environment and prevent new lesions from developing.

Logically, contemporary methods which minimise some of these risks should improve outcomes.

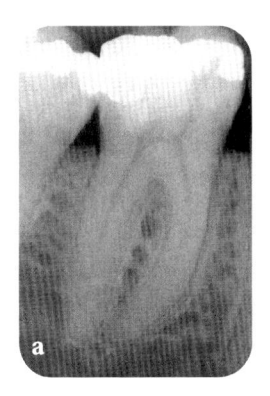

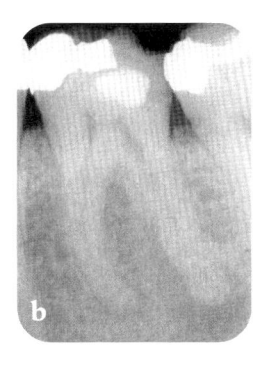

Fig 8-2 (a) Root canal treatment of this tooth is more likely to be successful in terms of periapical health at review than **(b)**.

Success and Failure

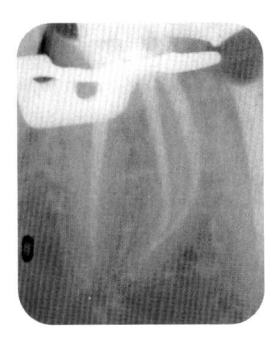

Fig 8-3 A root canal treatment expected to succeed, filled to within 2mm of root-end and with no real evidence of porosity. But this assumes all was done well. If the filling incorporated saliva, it may perform less well than a less aesthetically pleasing one packed in a clean canal.

Management and Maintenance of the Tooth after Treatment

Postoperative restoration
A well carried out root filling is no guarantee of painless, life-long function and periapical healing if the tooth and root filling are not immediately protected.

Root canal treated teeth can fail because of:
- fracture
- reinfection or entry of nutrient fluids from the mouth.

An adequate coronal restoration protects against both eventualities.
- For posterior teeth, that can be as simple as a cuspal coverage amalgam or composite restoration, extended well into the root canals, and bonded with a contemporary adhesive system (Fig 8-4).
- Temporary post crowns are especially vulnerable to coronal microleakage (Fig 8-5). Ideally, an anterior tooth should be sealed with a simple coronal plug until a cast post is ready for cementation, or a direct post/core provided immediately after root canal treatment. Crowns should provide wrap-around protection of tooth tissue to guard against fracture.

- Post space preparation is frequently associated with root weakening and perforation; two prominent causes of failure (Fig 8-6). Consensus is growing that posts should be used only when necessary to support and retain coronal restorations.
- Protective and well-sealing plastic restorations can serve adequately for many years, but definitive protecting and sealing restorations should not be unduly delayed if the tooth remains vulnerable to loss for non endodontic reasons.

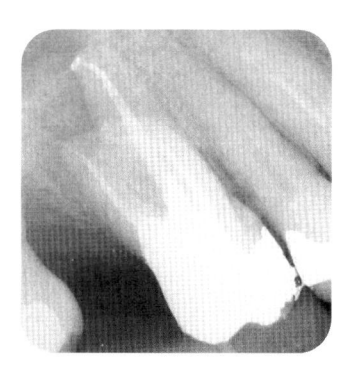

Fig 8-4 A well-conducted interim plastic restoration extended well into the canals for coronal seal and affording cuspal protection. (Courtesy G V Seccombe).

Ongoing maintenance
Pulpless teeth are as vulnerable to caries as any other. They are unlikely to become sensitive if recurrent caries develops, and lesions can quietly destroy the crown and reinfect the canal system if there is inadequate surveillance (Fig 8-7). Bisecting angle radiographs may not detect early coronal caries or marginal restoration breakdown.

Assessing Success and Failure from Different Perspectives at Intervals after Treatment

Immediately after closure of the tooth
Immediately after treatment, patients have few terms of reference to define success. Mild discomfort is usually no indicator of eventual outcome, and all patients should be advised to expect minor symptoms which may require simple analgesics for a few days.

Terms of reference are clearer for the clinician, who will judge his outcome and likelihood of pain relief and periapical healing on the basis of his knowledge of:

- what he did
- any serious procedural errors or compromises
- the radiographic appearance of the root filling.

Depending on the healthcare system, fee-paying authorities may make their judgement on the outcome based purely on the immediate postoperative radiographic appearance of the radiopaque white lines in the root canals (Fig 8-8). None demands to see evidence of successful healing.

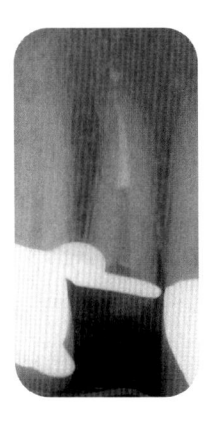

Fig 8-5 Temporary anterior post crowns – especially vulnerable to coronal microleakage. Ideally, the root would be sealed with a simple cement plug until a cast post was ready, or a direct post/core provided immediately the root canal treatment is complete.

Within one week of treatment
Effective treatment should have:
- eliminated or substantially reduced pain and swelling
- closed sinus tracts
- restored chewing function.

The patient's fee should have been paid, indicating satisfaction and no serious complaints. Occasionally, minor clinical symptoms persist after one week, but should be fully resolved within one month.

At this point, the patient may regard the treatment as a complete success with an expectation of symptom-free function for life. Depending on practice circumstances, clinicians may argue strongly that a successful outcome has been achieved, and make no further review of the case to check on the more stringent parameter of periapical healing or maintenance of health.

Within six months of treatment
Success may be inferred by:
- no unscheduled patient attendances
- the absence of symptoms or symptom-free signs of inflammation at recall.

When Should Periapical Healing be Reviewed Radiographically?

Guidelines suggest that unless there are:
- signs or symptoms of concern
- foundations are being checked for definitive reconstruction

there is no value in radiographic review until one year post-operatively Films at six months may give some indication of improvement, but transient lesions

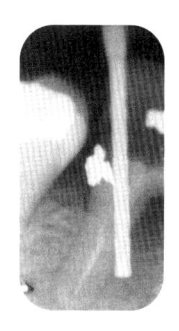

Fig 8-6 Catastrophic post space preparation – a common cause of failure and good reason to avoid posts unless needed.

can develop in response to debris pushed apically during treatment, which will resolve by one year.

One year after treatment
Clinical signs and symptoms which have emerged one year after treatment indicate that the case is failing, and that further care is needed after evaluation and discussion with the patient.

By this time:
- Approximately 90% of the periapical lesions which are going to heal will show clear signs of improvement, and 50% will have completely healed.
- Lesions which have diminished in size may be expected to continue healing unless new factors such as recurrent caries or loosening of a post-crown intervene.
- Lesions which appear to be unchanged are not necessarily failing, but are questionable and should be reviewed in a further twelve months. In the absence of new signs or symptoms, persistent lesions of this sort should be monitored for up to four years with annual radiographs. No further healing is likely after four years, and a final judgement can be made on whether the treatment succeeded or failed to prevent or heal apical periodontitis.

Why is Failure Important?

Persistence or development of symptoms (pain, discharging sinus, compromised chewing ability)
Failure to prevent or resolve symptoms is clearly recognised by patients who may seek remedy or recompense. Their case is less clear if symptoms develop several years after treatment rather than presenting symptoms failing to resolve or new symptoms emerging soon after treatment.

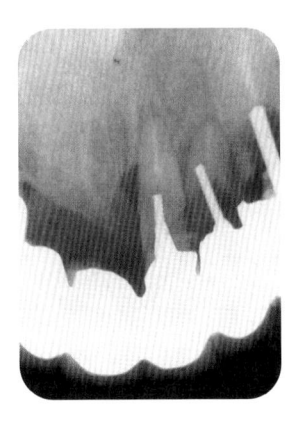

Fig 8-7 Silent destruction. Extensive caries has painlessly destroyed the crowns and reinfected the canal systems of these root canal treated teeth.

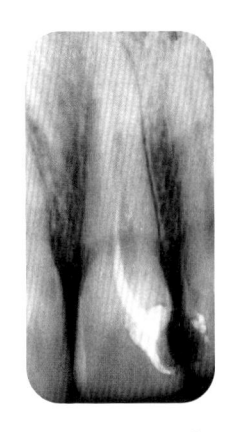

Fig 8-8 Success for the paymaster? Does this treatment justify the fee? Is it likely to achieve its desired goals?

It is foolish to offer 90% success rates to patients at the outset of treatment, since any compromise of infection control during or after treatment can impact seriously on prognosis. However, persistent pulpal and periapical symptoms are unlikely provided that all root canals are entered, prepared, filled and protected without serious procedural error.

Persistence of a periapical radiolucency
- The risk of acute flare-up. It is always a concern that persistent chronic lesions are flare-ups waiting to happen (Fig 8-9). The threat has never been properly quantified, but may involve 5% of teeth with chronic apical periodontitis in any year (i.e. 50% in a ten-year period). However, it is the experience of most dentists that these lesions are unpredictable, and most have witnessed the painful consequences at the most inopportune times. Interventions which upset the host–microbe equilibrium, such as replacing a restoration, are particularly likely to precipitate events.
- The potential threat of chronic infection. Links are becoming established between chronic marginal periodontitis and systemic disorders. Apical periodontitis is a similar, microbially mediated chronic inflammatory disease, and may pose similar threats. Patients may increasingly wish to see evidence that the treatment they receive cures them of the disease and eliminates other health risks, rather than simply suppressing overt symptoms.

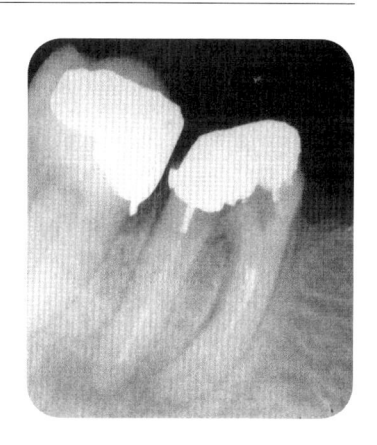

Fig 8-9 Persistent chronic apical periodontitis: what is the real risk of acute flare-up? Does any planned restorative work undermine confidence in this tooth remaining quiet?

We should all have an interest to audit the outcome of the care we prescribe and deliver. Clinical and radiographic follow-up is central to that process, and the failures we all encounter should translate into a review of our practices to control infection better and heal more lesions.

Conclusions

- Root canal treatment is effective in preventing and healing apical periodontitis, with success often quoted as 90%.
- The preoperative state, the treatment provided, and the management of the tooth after treatment, can seriously influence prognosis.
- There is little direct evidence to show which specific techniques treat apical periodontitis best.
- Patients, dentists and healthcare organisations should have an interest in ensuring that treatments heal disease, not simply produce pleasing radiographs or preserve a diseased status quo.

Further Reading

Consensus report of the European Society of Endodontology on quality guidelines for endodontic treatment. Int Endod J. 1994;27:115-124.

Friedman S. Treatment outcome and prognosis of endodontic therapy. In: Orstavik D, Pitt Ford TR (Eds.) Essential Endodontology. Prevention and Treatment of Apical Periodontitis. Oxford: Blackwell Science, 1998:367-401.

Murray CA, Saunders WP. Root canal treatment and general health: a review of the literature. Int Endod J 2000;33:1-18.

Index

A

Abscess *see also* apical periodontitis (symptomatic)
    Acute, principles of emergency management   13, 19
    Pulp   18
Accessibility for treatment, mouth opening   30
Accessory canals, secondary anatomy   61, 85, 97
Access   37, 51
    Calcified systems   51
    Cavity design   38
    Common errors   38, 50
    Principles   37
    Refinement for stress-free entry   47
    Safe-ended burs   46, 47
Acetaminophen (paracetamol)   22
Actinomyces   10
Ad pain fibres   14
Age changes, dentine/pulp complex   51
AHPlus   90, 97
Amoxicillin   23, 24
Anaesthesia,
    Failed   18
    Local   18, 31
Analgesics   13, 16, 22, 86, 117
Antibiotics   7, 13, 19, 22, 23, 24, 25
    Prophylactic   22, 30
    /Steroid preparation   19, 21, 62
Apex, open   106
Apex, gauging diameter   67, 72, 74, 77, 79, 81, 83
Apex locators, electronic   54, 68
Apexit   90
Apical calcification   53
Apical constriction   68
Apical control zone   74
Apical cysts, pocket and true   8
Apical enlargement
    Initial   70
    Final refinement (*see* Apex, gauging diameter)
Apical periodontitis
    Aetiology   3, 5-10
    Factors associated with treatment success   112
    Importance of treatment failure   119
    Prevalence   3
    Risk of flare-up   120
    Symptomatic, including emergency management   19-25
    Therapy resistant   8, 113
Apical pocket cyst   8
Apical trepanation   21
Apical true cyst   8
Articaine   19
Assessment, preoperative   27-31
Audit, of biological and healing outcomes from treatment   11, 121

B

Bacteria *see* microorganisms
Balanced Force instrumentation   65, 73
Blocked canals
    Non-calcified canals   58
    Tight and loose resistance   57
Burs
    Long, for chasing calcified canals   55
    Orientation during access   45, 50
    Selection for outlining access   45
    Safe-ended for unroofing pulp chambers   46

Index

C

Calcification	30, 51
And treatment compromise	51, 113
Apical	53
Reduction of pulp volume	52
Calcified inclusions	53
Entering calcified canal systems	54
Calcium hydroxide	
Non-setting	19, 21, 62
Root canal sealers	90
Canal preparation	59, 69
Engine-driven	75
Manual	70
Canine, access to the root canal	
Mandibular	43
Maxillary	40
Caries	4, 15, 16, 17, 19, 28, 117
Carrier obturation systems	104
Caulking, for rubber dam isolation	33
Cavit	33
Cavity outlines, classical	39
Cavity preparation	46
Cemento-dentinal junction	68
Central incisors, classic access	
Mandibular	43
Maxillary	39
C pain fibres	14, 17
Chlorhexidine	60, 62
Chronic infection, systemic consequences	3, 120
Clamps, for rubber dam isolation	32
Classical access cavity outlines	39
Cleaning and shaping	59
Clindamycin	23, 25
Compacted pulp tissue, blocking canal entry	58
Coronal access	37, 51
Coronal flaring	67, 70
Coronal seal	87, 108, 116
Cortical trepanation	21
Cracks, enamel/dentine	16, 29
Cross-sections, maxillary molar roots	43
Curving files, for canal negotiation	40, 57
Curvature	29
Treatment compromise and	29, 38, 62, 63, 113
Cuspal coverage restoration	31, 116
Customising gutta percha cones	92
Cyclic fatigue of rotary files	75
Cyst *see* Apical cysts	

D

Dam *see* Rubber dam.	
Decision-making	27
Dental caries *see* Caries	
Dentine bonding agents	17
Dentine-pulp complex	4
DG16 canal probe	42, 55
Diagnosis	13
Symptomatic pulpitis	14
Symptomatic apical periodontitis	19
Warning signs for hospital referral	25
Diamendo bur	46
Double-Flare canal preparation	70
Drainage	
Emergency	13, 18, 21, 24, 25
Incision and	22, 24, 25
Open, for persistent discharge	22
Drains	23
Dressings	
Coronal	17, 21, 108
intracanal	19, 21, 62, 86
Drugs *see* Antibiotics, Analgesics	
Drying, prior to root canal obturation	93

E

EDTA	57, 58, 61
Electronic apex locators *see* Apex locators	

Index

Electric motor 75
Electronic pulp testing 16, 20
Emergencies, endodontic 13
   see also specific conditions
Empirical prescribing 23, 24, 25
Endocarditis, infective 22, 30
Endo-Ray film holder 70
Endo Z bur 46
Engine-driven canal preparation,
   principles 75
Enlargement, passive prior to canal
   reparation 69
   see also Preparation, root canal
Enterococcus faecalis 10, 62
Erythromycin 23, 25
Ethyl chloride, soft-tissue anaesthesia 23
Extra-radicular infection 10

F

Feed of rotary files 75
File action
   Watch-winding 57
   Balanced Force 65
Files
   Curving for canal negotiation 57
   Hang-up during canal entry 53, 67
   ISO specifications 62
   Radial lands 64
   Tip design 64, 82
File systems 70, 73, 76
   GT manual 73
   GT rotary 87
   .06 systems (Profile, K3) 78
   642 systems (HERO, Flex-
      master) 79
   Progressive taper systems
      (ProTaper) 81
   Taperless systems (Lightspeed) 82
Film holders, for X ray exposures 70
Flare-up, risk in chronic apical perio-
   dontitis 120
Flaring, during canal preparation
   Coronal 67, 70
   Apical third 71
Flight path, stress free 38, 47
Flora
   Of diseased root canal system 4, 7, 9
   Disinfectant-resistant 8, 113
   Extra-radicular 8
Flexmaster 76
Flute loading, during apical
   preparation 72
Focal sepsis, threat of chronic
   infection 120
Fracture *see* Cracks.
Furcal perforation 45, 55

G

Gates-Glidden drills 49, 70, 83
Glass-ionomer, root canal sealer 90, 97
Goose-neck bur 55
Gutta percha 89
   Cold compaction 91
   Cone fit 92
   Warm compaction 97

H

Hang-up of files during access 53, 67
Healing 87
   Monitoring 111
Heat, in pulp diagnosis 16
Heat source
   System B 101
   Touch 'n' heat 94, 100
HERO 76
Host defences 7
Hot pulp, anaesthetic challenges 18

I

Ibuprofen 22

Index

Ice sticks 15, 17
Immunocompromised patients 14, 22
Incision and drainage 22, 24, 25
Incisors
    Mandibular 43
    Maxillary 39
Infection control 1, 8, 29, 59, 87
    Failure of 8, 115
Initial apical enlargement 70
Injection-moulded thermoplastic
    gutta percha 100
Instruments, stress-free flightpath 38, 47
    see also individual file systems
Intracanal medicaments *see* Dressings, intracanal
Intraosseous anaesthesia 18
Intrapulpal anaesthesia 19
Irreversible pulpitis 17
Irrigants 60
Irrigation 60
Irrigation needles, safe-ended 61, 62
Irritants
    Pulp 4
    Periapical 5
Irritation dentine 52
Isolation *see* Rubber dam

K

Ketac-Endo 90, 97
K3 system 76
K-file 62, 65
    Initial opening with 69

L

Lateral canals *see* Accessory canals
Lateral condensation 91
Lateral incisor
    Mandibular 43
    Maxillary 40
Ledermix 19

Ledging canals 37, 62
    see also Transportation
Length determination
    Consequences of error with ISO
        instruments 74
    Electronic 68
    Radiographic 68
Lentulospiral paste filler 93
Local anaesthesia *see* Anaesthesia, local
Lightspeed 76, 82
Lightspeed Simplifill 82, 96
Linear calcification *see* Calcification, calcified inclusions
Local medicaments 19, 21, 59, 62, 87
Lubrication 57, 58, 77, 92
Luer-loc syringe 61

M

Magnification 54, 57
Maintenance, of root canal treated
    teeth 116
Management, emergency 13
Marginal integrity, coronal
    restorations 28
Marginal percolation 4
Master apical file determination 67, 72, 74, 77, 79, 81
Master apical rotary 83
Master cone fit 92
Mandibular teeth 43
Maxillary teeth 39
Medical considerations, in endodontic
    treatment planning 30, 112
Medicolegal responsibility,
    rubber dam 32
Metronidazole 24, 25
Microleakage, percolation 4, 108, 116
Microorganisms
    Impact on treatment outcome 113
    Nature in endodontic disease 7
    Role in pulp disease 4

Index

Role in periapical disease 5
Therapy resistant 8
Mineral Trioxide Aggregate 55, 106
Mirror, front silvered 54
Molars
   Mandibular 44
   Maxillary 41
Monitoring
   In emergencies 17, 22, 25
   Of treatment outcome 117
Mouth opening
   Limited in spreading symptomatic apical periodontitis 23
   Limited in endodontic treatment planning 30
Multiple-visit treatment 86

N

Necrosis, pulp 4
Nickel-titanium
   Access refinements for 47
   Condensing instruments 91, 102
   Preparation instruments 66
   Properties 66
   Pros and cons of rotary systems 84
   See also individual file systems.

O

Obtundent pulp dressings 19
Obturation 87
   Carrier systems 104
   Cold lateral condensation 91
   Ideal materials 88
   MTA 106
   Principles 87
   Role of filling components 89
   Simplifill 96
   Thermomechanical compaction 94
   Vertical condensation, multiple wave 99
   Vertical condensation, single wave 101
   Warm gutta percha techniques 97
   When to fill root canals 88
Occlusal adjustment 22, 31
Open apex 106
Open drainage 22
OraSeal 33
Orientation, during access 45
Overdenture abutment 28
Overextension, irrigant, prevention 61
Overfill, loss of apical control 70, 74

P

Pain
   Pulpal 14
      Aδ fibre mediated 14
      Anaesthesia and 18
      C fibre mediated 15
      Diagnosis 15
      Emergency relief 16, 17
      Poor localisation 15
      Referral 15
      Reproduction 15
   Periapical 19
      Emergency relief 20, 21, 22, 23
   Relief, as an indicator of endodontic success 111, 117, 119
Paper points 54, 93
Paracetamol *see* Acetaminophen
Paramonochlorophenol 62
Passive enlargement, initial canal opening 69
Patency 68
Pecking file motion 75
Perforation repair 54
Periapical health, conditions for 6, 59, 87, 111
   Following preparation alone 8, 87
   Need for root fillings to secure 87
Persistent apical periodontitis 120

Persistent root canal infection	8	Non-vital	4
Physiological apex	68	Pulpectomy	1, 18, 58
Premolars		Pulp injury and death	4
Mandibular	43	Pulp stones	53
Maxillary	41	Pulp testing	16
Preparation, root canal		Electronic	16, 20
Crown-down	67	Thermal	16, 20
Engine driven, principles	75	Pulpitis	
Manual, with ISO instruments	70	Diagnosis	15
Manual with GT files	73	Emergency management	16, 17
Principles	59	Irreversible	17
Problems of traditional	62	Reversible	16
Rotary		Symptomatic	15
GT	77	Pulpotomy	19
.06 taper systems	78	Pulp stones *see* Calcification,	
642 systems	79	calcified inclusions	
Progressive tapers	81	Purulent focus, drainage 13, 18, 21, 22,	
Taperless	82	24, 25	
Techniques	69		
Preparing for definitive treatment	27		
Preserving endodontic health	87	**Q**	
Probe DG16	55		
Probing of canal entrances	55	Quality	
Profile	76	of treatment and outcome	114
Pros and cons, NiTi rotary			
preparation	84		
Post crowns, temporary	30, 116	**R**	
Post space preparation	97, 105, 116		
Postoperative restoration	116	Radial lands	64
Postoperative warnings	86, 107	Radicular cyst *see* Apical cysts	
ProTaper	76	Radiographic film holders	70
Protection of root fillings	108	Radiographic definition of successful	
Pulp Canal Sealer	90	treatment	112
Pulp		Radiographic monitoring	117, 118,
Access	37	119, 120, 121	
Age changes	51	Radiographic review of treatment	
Anatomy	38, 61	outcome	118
Breakdown	4	Radiographs	28, 45, 70, 118
Calcification	51	And case review	118
Calcified inclusions	53	And orientation for access	45
Canal space, reduction	52	And working length	70
Exposure	4, 39, 46	Preoperative	45
Fundamental clinical biology	1	Referral for treatment	29
Infection	4	Referred pain	15

Index

Refinement of access cavities 47
Reinfection and treatment
   failure 8, 87, 116
ReokoSeal 90
Reproduction of pulp symptoms 15
Resin-based sealers 90
Resistance to file entry 53, 55, 57
Restorability
   Compromise during access 37, 50
   prognosis 28
Restorations 17, 28, 88, 108, 116
   And cuspal protection 116
   And infection control 87
   And long-term outcome 108, 116
Restorative materials, pulpal
   irritancy 4
Reversible pulpitis 16
Review of treatment outcome 117
Road map, pulp chamber floor 46, 55
Root canal filling 87
   see Obturation
Root canal preparation 59
   see Preparation, root canal
Root canal infection
   Elimination 29, 59
   Nature 7
   Prevention of recurrence 87, 116
Root canal irrigation see Irrigants,
   Irrigation.
Root canal sealers
   Materials 90
   Application 93
Root canal systems
   Access 37
     see also individual teeth.
   Age changes 51
   Anatomy 37, 51
   Cleaning 59
   Complexity 60
   Disinfection 59
   Mechanical enlagement 59
   Persistent infection 8, 120
   Sealing 87
   Uninstrumented recesses 61, 85
Root filling see Obturation

Rotary root canal preparation 75
   see Preparation, root canal, also
     individual systems
Rotational, Balanced Force
   cutting 65, 73
Rotational speed and feed 75
Rubber dam
   Advantages of 32
   Application 33
   Clamp selection 32
   Indications 32
   Isolation 32
   OraSeal 33
   Sealing 33
   Slit-dam 33
   Wedjets 32, 35

S

Safe-ended access burs 46, 55
   Diamendo bur 46
   Endo Z bur 46
Scaler, ultrasonic 55
Sclerosed canals see Calcification
Seal
   Coronal 108, 116
   Root canal 87
   Rubber dam 33
Sealapex 90
Sealers 90
Sealer shoots 100, 105
Secondary anatomy see accessory
   canals
Sepsis, life threatening 13, 23, 25
Silicone-based sealers 90
Simplifill 83, 96
Single visit treatment 86, 114
Sinus 88, 112
Slit dam see Rubber dam
Smear layer 61
Snap-a-Ray film holder 70
Socio-economic considerations in
   planning 31

129

Index

Sodium hypochlorite 35, 50, 54, 58, 60
Softcore 104
Soft tissue incision 22, 24, 25
Speed of rotation 75
Speed reduction handpiece 75
Stepdown preparation 70
Steroid/antibiotic paste 19, 21, 62
Successful treatment
    Assessment 117
    Definitions 111
    Factors associated with 112
Supportive therapy 22, 25
Swelling
    localised 20, 22
    spreading 23
Symptomatic apical periodontitis 19
    Contained 20
    Spreading 23
Symptomatic pulpitis 15
    Irreversible pulpitis 17
    Reversible pulpitis 16
Symptoms, of endodontic disease 13
    After root canal treatment 119
Systemic disorders and apical
    periodontitis 3, 120

T

Tapered instrument systems 76
    see Preparation, root canal
Temperature
    Increased in emergencies 23, 25
    Influence on irrigants 60
Therapy resistant lesions 8
Thermafil 104, 106
Thermal pulp sensitivity 15, 16
Thermal pulp testing 15, 16
Thermomechanical compaction 94
Thermoplastic obturation.
    see Obturation, Warm gutta
    percha techniques
Tracking instrument use 76
Transportation 38, 63, 71, 72
Impact on infection control 63, 115
    Reducing 63
Traumatic occlusion 22, 31
Treatment
    Single or multiple visit 86
    Root canal, principles 1
Treatment outcome *see* Successful
    treatment
Treatment planning 27
Trepanation
    Apical 21, 22
    Cortical 21
Tooth Sleuth 16
Torque control motors 75
TubliSeal 90

U

Ultrasonic condensation 94
Ultrasonic scaler 55
Ultrasonic tips, cutting 57
Ultrasound
    Application of sealer cement 93
    Cutting dentine in canal location 57
    Disruption of pulp stones 55
    Irrigant activation 61, 85

V

Variably tapered instruments 81
Vegetable matter and apical
    periodontitis 10, 22
Vertical condensation
    Multiple wave 99
    Single wave 101
Vitality testing of pulp 15

W

Warm condensation techniques 97
Warm salt water mouthwashes 23

Watch-winding	57	**Z**	
Wedjet	32, 35		
Wedging device, crack detection	16	Zinc oxide-eugenol cements	
When to fill root canals	88	Dressing in symptomatic pulpitis	17
Working length	68, 70	Root canal sealer	90

X

X-ray film holders　　　　　69

Quintessentials for General Dental Practitioners Series

in 36 volumes

Editor-in-Chief: Professor Nairn H F Wilson

The Quintessentials for General Dental Practitioners Series covers basic principles and key issues in all aspects of modern dental medicine. Each book can be read as a stand-alone volume or in conjunction with other books in the series.

Publication date, approximately

Oral Surgery and Oral Medicine, Editor: John G Meechan

Practical Dental Local Anaesthesia	available
Practical Oral Medicine	Spring 2004
Practical Conscious Sedation	Autumn 2003
Practical Surgical Dentistry	Spring 2004

Imaging, Editor: Keith Horner

Interpreting Dental Radiographs	available
Panoramic Radiology	Autumn 2003
Twenty-first Century Dental Imaging	Autumn 2004

Periodontology, Editor: Iain L C Chapple

Understanding Periodontal Diseases: Assessment and Diagnostic Procedures in Practice	available
Decision-Making for the Periodontal Team	Autumn 2003
Successful Periodontal Therapy – A Non-Surgical Approach	Autumn 2003
Periodontal Management of Children and Adolescents	Autumn 2003
Periodontal Medicine in Practice	Spring 2004

Implantology, Editor: Lloyd J Searson

Implants for the General Practitioner	available
Managing Orofacial Pain in General Dental Practice	Spring 2003

Endodontics, Editor: John M Whitworth

Rational Root Canal Treatment in Practice	available
Managing Endodontic Failure in Practice	Autumn 2003
Managing Dental Trauma in Practice	Autumn 2003
Managing the Vital Pulp in Practice	Autumn 2004

Prosthodontics, Editor: P Finbarr Allen

Teeth for Life for Older Adults	available
Complete Dentures – from Planning to Problem Solving	Autumn 2003
Removable Partial Dentures – A Systematic Approach	Autumn 2003
Fixed Prosthodontics for the General Dental Practitioner	Autumn 2003
Occlusion: A Theoretical and Team Approach	Autumn 2004

Operative Dentistry, Editor: Paul A Brunton

Decision-Making in Operative Dentistry	available
Applied Dental Materials in Operative Dentistry	Spring 2003
Aesthetic Dentistry	Autumn 2003
Successful Indirect Restorations in General Practice	Spring 2004

Paediatric Dentistry/Orthodontics, Editor: Marie Therese Hosey

Child Taming: How to Cope with Children in Dental Practice	Spring 2003
Paediatric Cariology	Autumn 2003
Treatment Planning for the Developing Dentition	Autumn 2003

General Dentistry and Practice Management, Editor: Raj Rattan

The Business of Dentistry	available
Risk Management in General Dental Practice	Spring 2003
Practice Management for the Dental Team	Autumn 2003
Application of Information Technology in General Dental Practice	Spring 2004
Quality Assurance in General Dental Practice	Autumn 2004
Evidence-Based Care in General Dental Practice	Spring 2005

Quintessence Publishing Co. Ltd., London